WIN
THE
FAT
WAR

140 REAL-LIFE
SUCCESS STORIES

ANNE ALEXANDER

and the Editors of **PREVENTION** Health Books™

RODALE®

This edition first published in the UK in 2003 by
Rodale Ltd
7–10 Chandos Street
London W1G 9AD
www.rodale.co.uk

Printed and bound in the UK by The Bath Press

A CIP record for this book is available from the British Library
ISBN 1–405–00670–6

**This paperback edition distributed to the book trade by
Pan Macmillan Ltd**

Notice
This book is intended as a reference volume only, not as a medical manual. The information given here is designed to help you make informed decisions about your health. It is not intended as a substitute for any treatment that may have been prescribed by your doctor. If you suspect that you have a medical problem, we urge you to seek competent medical help.

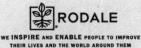

*To the many friends and readers
who helped me win the fat war.*

CONTENTS

ACKNOWLEDGEMENTS

This book owes a tremendous debt of gratitude – and, indeed, its origin – to the thousands of women and men who have shared their personal stories so that others can enjoy happier, healthier lives. I am grateful to all of the contributors for their honesty, authenticity and willingness to reveal their journeys, including their dark turning points as well as the secrets that created their personal triumphs and successes. Thank you for blazing a path so that others may follow.

My sincere thanks to my editor and friend, Debora Yost, for turning this book from an idea into 224 pages of paperback reality, with seemingly endless energy, enthusiasm and revisions that made it better every time. Thanks also to Michele Stanten, fitness editor at *Prevention* magazine, for her time and her dedication to providing the highest quality weight-loss information and advice both in this book and in every issue of the magazine. Additional thanks to Susan Berg, who edited, shepherded and nursed this project through its long and winding path.

Many other people had a hand in making this book a reality. For their hard work and grace under pressure, special thanks go to Susan Shelly McGovern, Doug Dollemore, Bridget Doherty, Judith Springer Riddle, Diane Gardiner Kozak, Eric Metcalf, Debra L. Gordon, JoAnne Czarnecki, Margo Trott, Linda Formichelli, Therese Iknoian, Linda Mooney, Staci Ann Sander and Jennifer Bright.

INTRODUCTION

I WON THE FAT WAR – AND YOU CAN, TOO

Congratulations! By picking up this book, you've taken the first step in a very important personal journey towards creating the life you want, free of the struggle with excess pounds, that constant battle between how you *want* to look and feel and what you see in the mirror every day.

We all come to this starting point from a different place. Maybe you're just sick and tired of feeling bad about the way you look. Maybe your doctor said that you have to get serious about your weight. Maybe you've just ridden that weight-loss roller coaster – up, up, up in pounds, down with a crash, then back up even higher next time – once too often and you want to get off for good.

Well, you can. You *can* win the fat war. Why am I so sure? Because I've been there and I won my own battle of the bulge. After nearly 10 years of being at war with my body, I finally called a cease-fire. No, I never weighed 21 stone. Instead, like a lot of men and women, my battle was with about 1½ stone, and most of it was waged in my head. (For those of you more accustomed to the metric system, 10 pounds is roughly 4.5 kg and 1 stone is roughly 6.5 kg, so use this as your guideline throughout.)

At age 13, I discovered cellulite on my thighs and decided that I needed to lose weight *pronto*. I also made the naïve calculation that if I could change my thighs – and my body weight – I would be happy (that is, self-confident, wildly popular, all of the magic that we associate with being thin). The result was that food became the focus of my life: reward, comfort, companion, even punishment. In a way, it was simple. A "good" day was when I'd eaten only a few morsels and gallons of diet fizzy drinks; a "bad" day meant that I'd slipped (how could I not?) and gorged on something from my endless list of "forbidden" foods. Instead of enjoying my life, I was focused on inane trivia like how my jeans fitted at that particular nanosecond. It was a vicious cycle and a total waste of time.

Finally, after years of inner turmoil and fluctuating weight, I decided to seek the help of a supportive counsellor and group of similarly obsessed women. Just meeting others who shared the same weight issues helped me see that I was far from alone.

One of the most important lessons that I learned was how to break my habit of focusing on food instead of solving the real, underlying problem. My counsellor taught me how to catch myself with the simple phrase *"Stop. Slow down and think."* When I was rushing out for a box of doughnuts, this phrase would pop into my mind, and I would pause long enough to figure out what was really bothering me. Once I'd got to the real source of my frustration, the doughnuts became much less important. It's a simple idea, but it does the trick for me. Today, I'm pleased to report, my weight is healthy, low and blessedly stable.

My experience with weight loss, however, was life-changing. Since then, I've been something of a crusader for healthy living. Having struggled for so long, I know what life is like on both sides – on and off the battlefield – and that it's entirely possible to win the fight once and for all.

I also know that winning isn't easy. Sometimes, it's hard work. You need to hear kind and encouraging words from people who've been in exactly the same boat, to know that they've felt just as lousy as you're feeling and to know that they managed to turn things around and become who they wanted to be. Well, here are 140 people to tell you how they did just that.

During my years as editor-in-chief of the world's largest health magazine, one of my greatest pleasures was hearing success stories from readers – letters and e-mails resounding the pride and pleasure of people who finally felt really good about themselves and wanted to share the seemingly miraculous news that they had finally lost weight. They could run, jump, play on the floor with the kids, wear sexy clothes, feel entitled to do whatever they wanted.

In fact, that's the reason that I decided to create this book – to share their victories and strategies so that together we can benefit from their success. We can benefit from the inspiration and motivation that comes from knowing that, yes, when you really set your mind to it, good things *do* happen. You *can* lose weight and learn to love your body. As you'll see, their stories are filled with important life lessons for all of us.

These winners are no different from you. They're all real people, and all of them generously agreed that we could use their real names. That's a testament to their courage, because many have revealed very important personal details about their struggles and setbacks as well as their victories. But they offered to tell their full stories because they know that their honesty can truly help *you* as you make your own decisions and take the actions that are right for you.

No matter what challenges we face as individuals, I believe that all of us can use some guidance and inspiration at the beginning. To help you get started on the right foot, I've summed up these guiding principles in the "Ten Commandments of Weight Loss" in the very first chapter of this book. From the thousands of success stories that I've heard, as well as my personal experience, I am convinced that these commandments are the most important when you're trying to reach your weight-loss goals.

But I also recognise that each of us faces our individual,

personal challenges. That's why I've divided the success stories into chapters that will speak most directly to you. As you'll see from their titles, the chapters focus on eating healthfully ("Feed Your Body Right"), your relationship with food ("End Emotion-Driven Eating"), exercise ("Get Your Body Moving"), self-image ("Feel Good About You") and motivation ("Stimulate Your Determination"). If you're not sure where to begin, you might think about the issue that has been most daunting to you in the past. Maybe the stories in that chapter are the ones you want to read first!

While each story in and of itself is unique, they all share a common bond. For each person, there was a single thing – a personal experience or diet trick – that made them turn the corner to their success. These are the "Winning Actions" that you'll find featured at the end of each story. I've added my own commentary to these Winning Actions because I believe there are ways that each of us can use these actions or learn something from them as we pursue our own journeys to success.

Now – just listen to the triumphs of these winners, and let yourself be filled with possibility. All you have to do is decide that, today, you want to win the fat war.

So turn the page and embark on creating your new life.

Anne Alexander

TEN COMMANDMENTS OF WEIGHT LOSS

The Ten Commandments that Moses brought down from Mount Sinai can keep you on the straight and narrow in your journey through life. In much the same way, the Ten Commandments of Weight Loss can guide your weight-loss efforts and show you the way to a healthier, happier lifestyle. They'll help you get started, and they'll serve as guideposts on your personal path to success.

As you go along, some of the Ten Commandments may become more important to you than others. That's okay. Use them for inspiration and motivation.

1 BELIEVE IN YOURSELF

Close your eyes and take a few quiet minutes to think about what has brought you to this point in your life. Think about the reasons why *you* want to slim down, not why other people want you to. This decision is about making yourself happy, not about making others happy. Real motivation can come only from inside you.

Maybe you want to have more energy so you can go cycling with your spouse or keep up with your kids. Maybe you want to avoid the health problems that have affected your parents or siblings. Maybe you're just tired of putting yourself down and you want to start feeling good about yourself.

Whatever reasons you come up with, write all of them down.

Keep your list somewhere you'll see it often. Tape it on your medicine cabinet or attach it to the fridge. Make a copy of it for your wallet and one for your office. Read it whenever you have a few minutes. Add new reasons as you think of them.

Every time you look at your list, reaffirm your decision to lose weight. Congratulate yourself for choosing to be good to yourself. Remember that you're leaving old, unhealthy habits behind and that you're creating a new future for yourself.

Once you make the decision to feel better, to live a happier, healthier life, and to take just as good care of yourself as you do of others, you *will* succeed. Believe in yourself. Thousands of others have won the fat war. You can, too!

2 SET THE RIGHT GOALS

Goals can keep you motivated and moving in the right direction – if you set the right ones. But how do you know what goals to set, and how do you make them realistic?

The first rule is to start small. Establish daily or weekly mini-goals to change some aspect of your behaviour that's standing between you and weight-loss success. It can be as simple as eating unsugared popcorn while you watch TV, instead of your usual bag of crisps. Or walking your kids to school every morning, rather than loading them into the car.

As you start to feel better, you'll naturally be inspired to set loftier goals. You may decide to give up crisps completely or to increase your walking time to a half-hour or even an hour a day. It's good to keep updating your goals as you make progress, but be sure to keep them doable.

The second rule of goal setting is to write down your goals. Seeing them in front of you takes them from the abstract and makes them real. I have a friend who writes her goals on Post-It notes and sticks them on her bathroom mirror. They're the first thing that she sees every morning, and they remind her of her new priorities.

However you choose to do it, keep your goals manageable and visible. Stick with them and watch them work!

3 EAT MORE

Eat more to weigh less? Absolutely! You can heap your plate with juicy, sweet, wonderful-tasting fruits; colourful, crunchy vegetables; and filling, satisfying grains. Slimming down does *not* mean being hungry or skipping meals or living on iceberg lettuce and sticks of celery.

You not only can eat more, you can eat more often. Studies have shown that switching from two or three large, heavy meals to five or six healthy mini-meals keeps your metabolism revved up and burning calories. It also keeps your energy level high, so you're always ready to get up and move around.

Make your meals interesting and enticing. Try fruits and veggies that you have never had before. Many supermarkets now carry a selection of exotic produce like star fruits, papayas, clementines, kale and Swiss chard. Experiment with herbs, spices, flavoured vinegars and other condiments that add tons of flavour with little fat and few calories.

Food is not the enemy when you're trying to lose weight. It's your ally. Choose wisely, and you will become slimmer, healthier and more energized.

4 EAT SMART

Eating more can help you realise your weight-loss goals. But you have to be smart about it. If you coat your wonderful lunch salad with a high-fat dressing, it's not so wonderful anymore. If you load your whole-grain roll with butter, it topples out of the healthy category and into the not-so-healthy one.

The easiest and fastest way to teach yourself to eat intelligently is to keep a food diary. In a small notebook, write down exactly when, what and how much you eat. Was the fish grilled or fried? Did you have one serving of ice cream, or two . . . or three? Was your baked potato topped with plain low-fat yogurt and chives or with butter and sour cream?

You may be surprised at how your perception of what and how much you eat differs from what really goes into your mouth. You may never have realised how many handfuls of M&M's you grab from the office sweet bowl over the course of a day. Or that the bottle of cola that you drink with your lunch contains two servings rather than one. Or that your usual-size portion of fish is three times larger than it should be. All of those extra calories add up.

Learn to recognise portion sizes. Weigh and measure foods until you know what a serving looks like. And always read labels. You'll be amazed at where you'll find loads of calories lurking.

Eating smart isn't about eating boring, tasteless meals – or not eating at all. It's about eating only when you're hungry, making healthy food choices, and controlling your portions. It's about being aware of why you're eating. It's about feeding your body properly and feeling good about yourself.

▮5 GET MOVING

An active lifestyle is extremely important for everyone, regardless of whether they want to lose weight. Time and again, studies have shown that those who exercise regularly tend to live longer and feel more satisfied with themselves than those who never get off the sofa. Just think of the people that you know. Chances are that those who get out and move around regularly are more energetic and vital than those who don't.

If you're just launching an exercise programme, the important thing is to start slowly. Five minutes of something as simple as walking is enough at first, especially if you've been inactive. Just increase the length of your walks by about 5 minutes a week, until you're getting 45 to 60 minutes of exercise at least 5 days a week.

This doesn't mean that you need to spend all of that time on a treadmill or stairclimber. There are dozens of activities that can provide an aerobic workout. The choice is up to you. Dust off your old 10-speed bike and go for a ride. Play tennis or sign up for an aqua-aerobics class. Find an activity that you enjoy. That way, you'll be more likely to stick with it.

Also, try varying your exercise routine so that it doesn't become tedious. If you ride an exercise bike for 45 minutes on Monday, go for a walk in the woods on Tuesday. Or take your bike outside on the patio for a change of scenery. Once in a while, throw in an activity that you've never done before, like rock climbing or rollerblading or tai chi.

And don't overlook the little things that you can do to enhance your health and fitness – and burn a few extra calories. Instead of driving around the supermarket car park three times, looking for the space closest to the door, leave your car out in the hinterlands. Clean out the garage, rake up the leaves in the garden or hang the laundry outside rather than using the dryer.

Over time, activity and exercise will become a natural, even enjoyable part of your life. Have faith and give it a try.

6 BUILD MUSCLE

While aerobic exercise revs up your metabolism and improves your level of fitness, it's strength training that builds muscle. That's important because the more muscle you have, the higher the rate at which your body burns calories. What's more, muscle burns more calories round the clock, even when you're curled up on the sofa reading a good book.

Can't imagine yourself walking into a gym and inquiring where you might find the weight room? Then do a simple but effective strength-training programme in your own home, using hand weights or even soup tins. Still, you may want to consult a personal trainer, who can teach you a routine as well as proper form.

A 15- to 20-minute session, 2 or 3 days a week, is all the strength training that you need to build muscle and develop a sleeker, firmer appearance. And you'll see results in as little as 6 to 8 weeks. You'll feel stronger and more confident. Your clothes will fit better. Your belly will be flatter; your arms and legs, more toned and shapely.

So go ahead and start lifting. You'll love what you see – and how you feel.

7 BINGE-PROOF YOUR LIFE

If you're prone to bingeing, don't worry. You *can* stop it and take control of your eating habits. But first you must understand why it happens. What sorts of things cause you to overeat? For some people, the cause is stress, loneliness, anger or sadness. For others, it's dining out with friends, going on holiday or having a good time at a party.

Reading your food diary can help you recognise and antici-pate the emotions or situations that lead to your binges. As you become more aware of what's setting you off, you can avoid those situations and find other, non-food sources of comfort.

If you feel that you are heading for a binge or if you catch your-self in the middle of one, you can still stop it. Simply walk away – leave everything where it is and get out of the house. A brisk walk around the block can give you time to think about what's making you want to eat. Once you get back home, you'll have a new per-spective on the situation, and you may realise that you're not interested in eating after all.

There may be times when you're nursing a craving – say, for chocolate mocha almond ice cream – that you have no choice but to go ahead and help yourself. Not to a huge bowl, mind you. And definitely not to the whole carton. Scoop out a single serving and put the rest back in the freezer. Then really *enjoy* that ice cream. Let each spoonful melt in your mouth and wash over all of your tastebuds.

When worse comes to worst and you indulge in an all-night bingefest, don't berate yourself afterwards. You have to accept what happened and move on. There's no point in kicking yourself because you messed up. Just be sure to add a half-hour to your next workout, and be extra careful about what you eat for the next few days.

8 TALK YOURSELF THIN

If one person on a weight-loss programme is good, then one person with a partner must be better, right? In most cases, the answer is yes.

A buddy can be an encourager, a confidante, a co-conspirator and a calming influence. She can persuade you to put on your walking shoes and go for a stroll when you'd rather be vegging out in front of the TV or pigging out on fast food. She'll listen attentively when you confess to eating a whole bag of chocolate-chip biscuits, then suggest that the two of you play a couple of sets of tennis that afternoon.

So how do you go about recruiting someone for this all-important position? Use some common sense, and trust your instincts. If you regularly run into trouble at the office when people bring in cakes and biscuits, consider asking the person at the next desk to be your morale booster. If you need someone to coax you out of bed for your 6:00 a.m. workout, maybe your spouse is the weight-loss partner for you.

Nobody at home with you? Look on the Internet. There are all kinds of weight-loss chat rooms, including those connected with the websites of organisations such as Weight Watchers.

Once you think that you've found your weight-loss buddy, tell that person what you expect. Are you looking for moral support? A workout partner? Somebody to talk to when the going gets tough? Make your wants and needs clear. That's the only way that your buddy can help you.

9 MAKE MOTIVATION EASY

When you first get serious about slimming down, it's easy to feel motivated. And it's a real high when you start to see results.

But after you've been plugging away at your weight-loss programme for a while, it can feel a little old. Maybe you find yourself thinking, "What the heck, one doughnut won't hurt anything." Or maybe your workouts are getting on your nerves – they take up too much of your time or they're boring. Or maybe you've reached a plateau and you haven't lost so much as an ounce in weeks.

What do you do when you hit the weight-loss skids? You jump-start your motivation, that's what.

Get out your list of reasons why you want to slim down, and remind yourself of your purpose. Remember what you weighed when you started, and note how many pounds you've lost. Count how many more minutes you can walk or run or swim. Congratulate yourself on the job that you've done so far, and adjust your goals to get you where you want to be. Be sure to write them down and put them where you'll see them.

If you haven't lost any weight for a while, try to figure out why. Maybe those doughnuts and skipped workouts have something to do with it. But if you've been faithful to your original eating-and-exercise plan, it could be that you're burning fewer calories because you weigh less. A 11st 6lb body burns fewer calories during a 30-minute jog than a 13st 8lb body. In that case, you may have to cut your calorie intake a little more or work out a little longer to make up the difference.

Keep in mind that everyone hits plateaus when they're trying to lose weight. And lapses in motivation are perfectly normal. The trick is to overcome them and move on. You've come such a long way. Don't give up now!

🔟 REWARD YOURSELF

Remember when you were a kid and you brought home an excellent school report? You knew that your high marks would earn praise from your parents, and you looked forward to hearing what a good student you were. The money that you'd get from Grandpa wasn't bad, either.

All of us like to be recognised for what we do well. This is just as true when we're trying to lose weight as when we earned an "A" in arithmetic.

Some of the most memorable rewards that you receive will come from others. But even more important are the rewards that you give yourself.

Remember the first commandment, "Believe in yourself"? When you acknowledge each weight-loss goal that you have achieved, you are honouring the commitment and hard work that you've put into creating a new, healthier life for yourself. You don't have to wait for the big, "I-lost-75-pounds!" sort of goals, either. Something as small as adding an extra mile to your daily walk or not eating chips for a week can be cause for celebration.

So go ahead! Take a half-day off work. Go shopping. Get a manicure. Buy tickets for the theatre. Do something that you really love but don't usually make the time to do.

When you reward yourself for a job well done, you reinforce your belief in yourself and tell yourself that you're proud of what you've accomplished. It makes you want to do more, to see how far you can go. And that's what living life to the full is all about.

FEED YOUR BODY RIGHT

AN INSULT MADE HER FIT

A New Year's Eve party to welcome 1994 served as the wake-up call that Meredith Willson needed to get serious about slimming down.

"At the time, I weighed more than 21st 6lb," recalls the 43 year old. "Someone that I hadn't seen in years came up to me and said, 'What happened to the Meredith I used to know?' It was a shock – and shock therapy is a good way to get inspired."

The next day, Meredith set her sights on a rather lofty resolution: to lose 120 pounds in 12 months. It was ambitious, but Meredith was convinced that eliminating red meat and processed food from her diet would do the trick. "Cheese and butter were the toughest," she says. "Instead of giving them up completely, I switched to fat-free cheese and butter substitutes." She also began eating more fresh foods – fruits, vegetables and whole grains.

Meredith read cookbooks that taught her how to make the most of fresh ingredients in her cooking. She also planted a garden chock full of organic produce, including tomatoes, broccoli, marrows, asparagus and aubergines. "The closer you get to the ground, the better off you'll be, nutrient-wise," she says. Then, using her homegrown produce plus healthy staples from the supermarket, she spent time each weekend preparing food from scratch. She even made her own pasta, tomato sauce and baked sweet-potato crisps.

Even Meredith couldn't believe how well her switch from

processed foods to fresh worked. "I lost 12 pounds every month – ka-bam, ka-bam, ka-bam," she says. "I never even hit a plateau."

In just over a year, Meredith managed to take off 150 pounds. And she has maintained that weight loss ever since.

WINNING ACTION ➤➤➤

Take a fresh approach to eating. Fresh foods are naturally high in fibre and low in fat – the perfect weight-loss combination. Plus, they have more intense flavours, so you won't feel compelled to overeat. Among the best fresh foods for weight loss are potatoes, oranges, apples and grapes. Researchers have identified these as high-satisfaction foods, which means that they keep you full longer.

AT DINNERTIME, SHE DESERTS HER FAMILY

Make no mistake: Debbee Sereduck loves her husband and her three children. But for 3 years, she refused to eat dinner with them. Sacrificing a little family togetherness was tough, but it helped Debbee take off an astounding 234 pounds.

Debbee, aged 38, doesn't remember a time when she was thin. At 5 foot 11 inches, she carried her weight well – for a while. But the scales never seemed to stop climbing upwards. By the age of 33, she had reached 29st 8lb.

Self-conscious about her appearance and concerned about the effects that her weight might have on her health, Debbee felt that she had to slim down. She just couldn't get herself motivated to do it. That changed one day in 1994, when she turned on her television and saw rescue workers extricating a large woman from her home and placing her in a special van to take her to the hospital. "The reporter mentioned that the woman weighed 40 stone, and I was mortified," Debbee says. "That wasn't much more than I weighed."

With the image of the woman fresh in her mind, Debbee launched a self-styled weight-loss programme that consisted primarily of eating low-fat foods in more sensible portions and riding an exercise bike. "I knew what I had to do," she says. "I just needed the motivation to do it."

Exercising was tough at first because Debbee was so overweight and out of shape. "I'd just tell myself, 'I'm going to pedal that bike for as long as I can,'" she says. "I made myself sit on it for an hour every day, whether or not I was actually riding."

Debbee had an easier time adjusting her eating habits, but dinnertime remained a struggle. How could she eat a carefully portioned meal while watching her family help themselves to seconds? How could she just throw away perfectly good food that her kids didn't finish?

Rather than wrestle with these temptations, Debbee decided to walk away from them. Every evening, she prepared dinner and served it to her family. Then she took her meal into the living room and ate by herself. She didn't return to the kitchen or dining room until everything was cleaned up and put away. "This kept me from dipping into the serving bowls for extra helpings and from finishing off the kids' uneaten food," she says. "It also gave me a few minutes of peace and quiet."

Her strategy worked like a charm. Over the next 3 years, Debbee took off 234 pounds, reaching her goal weight of 12st 12lb. She has held steady ever since.

Were all of those dinners alone worth the effort? Debbee thinks so. Now that she's fit, she has even more opportunities to enjoy life with her family. "I used to be a very active person, but I hadn't been on a bicycle since I was 11 or 12. I really wanted to go riding with my kids, which we now do all the time," she says. "I'm able to do the kinds of things that I couldn't do before."

HALF HER BODY WEIGHT – GONE

At the age of 31, Pamela Joyce Kimrey had to face facts.

Her father had died of a massive heart attack when he was just 35 years old. Pamela Joyce wondered if the same fate awaited her. After a lifetime of overeating and almost 2 decades of yo-yo dieting, she weighed 19st 8lb. And she was scared.

Pamela Joyce traced her seemingly endless appetite to her childhood. "When I was born, I weighed a little more than 4 pounds," she explains. "My parents left the hospital with instructions to feed me as often and as much as they could." And they did. By the time she was 11 years old her weight hovered around 9st 4lb.

Through school, Pamela Joyce continued to gain. She left weighing close to 17st 12lb, far too much for her 5-foot-2-inch frame. "I didn't want to go through college overweight. I wanted to fit in," she recalls. "So I put myself on what I considered a diet. I ate less, but I ate poorly – mostly deep-fried, sugary and fatty foods." Over the next year, she took off 5 stone. "At 12st 12lb, I still weighed too much for my height," she says. "But I held steady for several years, right through my wedding in March 1987."

As Pamela Joyce settled into married life, the pounds started coming back. "Twenty-five pounds stuck around after I gave birth to our only child," she says. "The rest of the weight resulted from too many meals of fried food smothered in gravy, plus thousands of calories worth of junk food and fizzy drinks."

By October 1996, Pamela Joyce had reached her top weight of 19st 8lb. "One night, I was lying in bed, feeling disgusted with myself. I started thinking about my dad, and I realised that I could die young if I didn't take better care of myself. It was my wake-up call."

The very next day, Pamela Joyce went to her local library and took out every nutrition, fitness and weight-loss book that she could find. When she read them, she found three themes that came up over and over again: a low-fat diet with portion control, regular exercise and plenty of water.

Based on the information that she had collected, Pamela Joyce put herself on a strict 1,200-calorie-a-day diet. She cut out junk food, whole milk and butter and began grilling and baking food instead of frying it. She also invested in kitchen scales to keep tabs on portion sizes.

Because she was accustomed to eating as much as she wanted, Pamela Joyce had to find a way to keep her stomach full throughout the day. One of her favourite tricks was to save a part of each meal for later in the day. "If my breakfast consisted of a bowl of raisin bran, skimmed milk and a banana, I'd save the banana for a mid-morning snack," she explains. "Likewise, I'd keep half of my lunch sandwich for an afternoon snack. If I ate out, I'd have half of my main course wrapped to go before I'd even take a bite."

This strategy helped Pamela Joyce stay within her 1,200-calorie limit without feeling hungry. Between her improved eating habits, her daily workouts (alternating aerobic exercise and strength training) and her consumption of gallons of water a week, she managed to lose 137 pounds – exactly half of her body weight – in a little more than 2 years. She's been holding steady since November 1998.

"There is absolutely no way to compare the old me with the new me," Pamela says. "I could never have imagined how wonderful

I feel. I can keep up with my son and not worry about embarrassing him – except maybe when we're rollerskating in the park. Good health has become a way of life for me and my family."

WINNING ACTION ➤ ➤ ➤

Eat less more often. Three cheers for Pamela Joyce. What an incredible story! If you can't resist between-meal snacking, do what Pamela Joyce did and save part of a meal for later on. You'll never get too hungry, since you'll be feeding your body every few hours. Plus, you'll avoid taking in too many calories in one sitting.

---

95 POUNDS IN 1 YEAR: WEIGHT LOSS FOR THE RECORD BOOK

For Kelly Jens, food was once an all-consuming passion.

"I was always thinking about what my next meal would be," says the 28 year old. "When I'd go out to eat, I'd try to pick places with the biggest portions or the most courses. I especially liked Quarter Pounders with Cheese, nachos, pizza with extra cheese and anything with Alfredo sauce."

Always on the hefty side, Kelly couldn't stop eating – or stop gaining weight. By Christmas 1997, she had reached 15st 10lb. "In a picture with my husband and my two kids, my little 1-year-old looks like a doll in my huge lap," she recalls. "I thought to myself, 'I don't want my children to have a fat, unhealthy mother.'"

It was time to change her life.

Using information she gathered from *Prevention* magazine and books by weight-loss guru Richard Simmons, Kelly determined that she would need to trim her daily calorie intake to 1,400 in order to achieve and maintain a healthy weight.

Obviously, that was far fewer calories than she had been consuming. To help herself stay on course, she began keeping a food diary. Kelly would write down every morsel she ate and every drop she drank – usually before she ate or drank it. She also noted the calorie and fat content of each item.

To help herself burn calories, Kelly started using a Health Walker, a nonimpact machine that allows the legs to swing back and forth to simulate striding. At first, she worked out for 15 minutes per session, then gradually built up to an hour a day – a schedule that she still maintains. She also does strength training twice a week, exercises to a kickboxing video and skips.

In 1 year, Kelly lost 95 pounds. And the weight hasn't come back. For that, she credits her food diary. "I never really knew how much I was eating until I starting writing it down and reviewing it," she explains. "Even though I've learned what I can eat and how much, I still keep a diary. It's a good tool for helping me maintain my present weight."

WINNING ACTION ➤ ➤ ➤

Keep a diary. Buy a small spiral-bound notebook and carry it with you. Immediately after meals and snacks, write down what you've consumed, along with the food's fat and calorie content. Studies show that people tend to be more true to their diets when they keep a record of what they eat.

SUCCESS WITH AN INTERNATIONAL FLAVOUR

Three times a day, Alice Layne takes a trip around the world – not in an aeroplane, but on her plate. Her adventurous approach to eating helped her lose 67 pounds and four sizes within 2 years.

Alice, a 42 year old, didn't always have a daring palate. Growing up, she feasted on lots of pizza and sugar. "My mother's idea of a treat was a box of brown sugar cubes, a chocolate bar or a tub of ready-mixed icing," she says.

Alice's unhealthy food choices caught up with her during her teenage years, when she started gaining weight. Her eating habits didn't improve as she got older, either. A typical day featured a sugary cereal for breakfast, a bulky sandwich for lunch and dinner in a restaurant, where she'd eat to the point of discomfort.

By her late thirties, despite bouts of yo-yo dieting, Alice had reached 16st 11lb. Her waistline wasn't all that suffered. Her back ached due to her weight and her self-esteem tumbled.

"My breaking point came when I had to go away for a weekend and I ordered several new outfits for the trip," she says. "I didn't try on the clothes before leaving and when I got to where I was going, I discovered that nothing that I had bought fitted."

Hurting physically and emotionally, Alice knew that she had to slim down. Over the next year and a half, she made a modest effort to improve her eating habits, which led to a 23-pound weight loss.

At that point, she felt that she needed a programme with structure, so she joined Weight Watchers. Her group leader introduced her to international foods that made her meals more exciting and healthy.

Alice enticed her tastebuds with ethnic favourites that she found in cookbooks: tabbouleh, a minty wheat salad from the Middle East; couscous, a pebbly pasta from northern Africa; and polenta, a cornbreadlike food flavoured with roasted red peppers and tomatoes that's popular in Italy. Along the way, she learned how to cook with the salsas and spices that flavour many ethnic cuisines. "The new tastes transformed my palate," she says. "Now, when I take even a bite of some of the foods that I used to eat, I don't like them."

Alice had so much fun experimenting with exotic new recipes that she never felt like she was dieting. Yet she lost 44 pounds in less than 6 months, reaching her personal goal weight of 12 stone in December 1998. And she has held steady ever since.

Alice says that she seldom visits her chiropractor for her aching back anymore. And she feels much stronger emotionally, now that her self-esteem isn't bogged down by extra weight.

"Since I've slimmed down, I've had my hair cut and styled differently," she says. "Many people don't even recognise me, which is fun."

WINNING ACTION ➤ ➤ ➤

Explore the world via your dinner plate. Some of the healthiest low-fat meals come from other cultures. Tempt your tastebuds with Greek souvlakia (lamb served on skewers), French ratatouille (a vegetable dish cooked in olive oil), Japanese yakitori (grilled chicken), Thai ginger beef or Indian mulligatawny (a kind of lentil soup).

These are just a few examples of the "world's fare" that can please your palate without widening your waistline. Consider investing in ethnic cookbooks.

SHE TRAINED HER BRAIN TO SAY "WHEN"

Linda O'Hanlon used a measuring cup to lose 57 pounds.

Overweight since she was a child, Linda never developed that "I'm full" signal that makes most people push away their plates after eating a serving or two. "When I sat down for a spaghetti dinner, I didn't get up until every last strand of pasta in the pot was gone," she recalls.

Over the years, as her weight crept upwards, Linda invested a great deal of money in fad diets with hopes of slimming down. But they didn't help. "I'd lose 5 pounds and go off the diet," she explains. "Then I'd gain back the 5 pounds, plus another 5."

By the time Linda reached 14st 12lb, she gave up trying to lose weight, resolving to accept herself as she was. But that changed in August 1997, when she went with a friend to Weight Watchers. Through the programme's meetings, she learned how to make healthy food choices and control her portion sizes. "The lesson was that if you put junk in your body, you'll feel like junk," she says.

She took that lesson to heart. Realising that she had a natural tendency to overeat, Linda became extra-vigilant about her portion sizes. When she'd sit down for pasta, she'd pull out her trusty measuring cup and carefully measure out 1 cup of spaghetti, 1 cup of cooked vegetables and 1 cup of garden salad. She'd eat that and no more.

Over time, Linda became adept at eyeballing her portion sizes. By relying on her brain instead of her stomach to say "when," she dropped three trouser sizes in 7 months. Two years later, at the age of 30, she's holding steady at 10st 11lb. "My clothes fit great and I'm bursting with energy," she says.

WINNING ACTION ➤ ➤ ➤

Learn to recognise portion sizes. For foods that are easy to overdo, especially pasta, cereal and ice cream, measure out one serving and transfer it into the bowl you would normally use. Make a mental note of how it looks (it's probably a lot smaller than you're used to seeing). You'll need some time to retrain your brain, but eventually, the smaller portions will seem normal.

THIS WINNER RUNS TO EAT

When Rick Myers decided to slim down, he gave himself a choice. He would either consume fewer calories or burn more with exercise. He chose the latter and took off more than 50 pounds.

Rick, a 46-year-old barber, admits that he has a passion for eating. But until he joined Weight Watchers in 1990, he had never exercised. "I got the message right away that I couldn't lose weight and keep it off without working out," he says. "So a week after I joined, I started walking."

Back then, Rick weighed 17st 2lb. He could barely walk for 15 minutes without tiring. But he stuck with it, gradually working his way up to 45 minutes – about 3 miles – every day. By the end of that year, he had lost more than 50 pounds.

More than a year later, still buoyed by his success, Rick decided to step up his exercise programme. "I didn't want to worry about every little thing that I ate," he explains. "I figured that if I switched from walking to running, I'd burn more calories." In fact, he started running the day that he successfully quit smoking, April 14, 1992.

"At first, I thought that by running, I could cut my workout time a little," Rick says. "But then I got addicted to running. My workouts were twice as long as when I was walking."

Now, Rick runs for about an hour every day, covering about 7 miles. He also goes to a gym three times a week.

While Rick's workouts may seem demanding, they're the price that he's willing to pay for the freedom to enjoy his favourite foods. "You have to strike a balance between the amount of food that you eat and the amount of exercise that you do to keep your weight pretty much the same," he says.

Rick's eating habits have improved, however. These days, he says that eating healthily and exercising regularly are as natural for him as overeating and smoking used to be. And those 50 pounds that he lost never came back. "My only regret is that I waited so long before making these changes," he says.

> **WINNING ACTION ➤ ➤ ➤**
>
> **Pick your battle plan.** Consume more calories than you burn and you'll gain weight. Consume fewer calories than you burn and you'll lose weight. It's that simple. You just have to decide whether you want to focus on reducing your calorie intake from foods or on burning more calories through exercise. Or if you want, focus on both. Just do what feels right for you.

SMALL CHANGES MADE A 147-POUND DIFFERENCE

A routine visit to the doctor totally changed Tammy Munson's life.

Tammy, 33, admits that she knew very little about good nutrition when she was younger. Even though she routinely ate high-fat foods such as chicken wings, pepperoni pizza and chips, she couldn't understand why she kept packing on the pounds. "I just didn't know any better," she says. By the age of 21, she weighed in at 18st 1lb.

Then, during a routine checkup, Tammy found out that she had alarmingly high blood pressure. The news jolted Tammy into action. Determined to slim down, she began paying more attention to her diet. She switched from full-fat milk and sugary drinks to skimmed milk and diet drinks – and lost 30 pounds. She had never considered how her beverage choices contributed to calorie intake. This surprised her so much that she decided to learn everything she could about healthy eating.

"I went to the library and signed out every nutrition book I could find," she says. "I was determined to make better food choices so that I could lose more weight." She also read dozens of cookbooks and discovered how to turn fat-laden recipes into nutritious meals with a few simple ingredient substitutions.

All of that reading transformed Tammy's eating habits. Within about a year, she lost a total of 147 pounds. And she has stayed at 7st 8lb ever since, thanks to 12 years of healthy eating.

WINNING ACTION ➤ ➤ ➤

Find out what you're really eating. For one day, write down everything that you eat and drink, along with the fat and calorie content of each item. At the end of the day, add up your numbers. Surprise! You're probably eating more than you realised.

SHE CUT HER PLATE IN HALF AND LOST 25 POUNDS

When it comes to cleaning her plate, Barbara Vaughan knows where to draw the line, quite literally. She has been doing it for 30 years.

Like most of us, Barbara learned at an early age not to waste food. "In my family, it was a sin to not finish everything on your plate," recalls the 51-year-old businesswoman. "I'd sit at the table for hours because my parents wouldn't allow me to leave until I'd eaten my peas. When you're raised like that, you get conditioned to clean your plate. It's a habit that's really hard to break."

Barbara's clean-plate habit stayed with her when she went to college, where the cafeteria served jumbo-size portions of practically everything. True to form, she ate every last bite. Her weight climbed to 10st 5 lb during her first year alone.

As the pounds piled on, Barbara grew more and more dissatisfied with her appearance. She knew that she was eating a lot more than she should and that the extra calories were contributing to her weight gain. So she set out to break herself of her clean-plate habit for good. And she used a knife to do it.

Whenever Barbara sat down to a meal in the campus cafeteria, she'd take her knife and draw a line right down the middle of her plate, bisecting the meat, the mashed potatoes or whatever else she was served. Then she ate only the food to one side of the line, leaving the rest behind. This simple trick cut Barbara's portions in half. It also enabled her to change her clean-plate mindset. "That line showed me when I had eaten enough," she explains. "I could let the rest of my food lie without guilt."

Her strategy worked. By the time Barbara graduated from college, she had taken off 25 pounds. She has maintained her weight at a healthy 8st 8lb ever since.

WINNING ACTION ➤ ➤ ➤

Draw the line on eating. One way to teach yourself portion control is to use Barbara's technique. Use your knife to draw a line right down the middle of your plate. Eat only the food to one side of the line and leave the rest. You can save it for another meal!

SHE LOST HER EATING "HABIT" AND 102 POUNDS

Robin Wade struggled with her weight for most of her adult life. Only when she learned to listen to her body did the pounds disappear.

Robin was raised on a diet of fried and gravy-smothered foods. Eventually, she turned her love of food and her talent for cooking into a successful career as a certified dietary manager, supervising restaurant kitchens.

The problem was that Robin got in the habit of taste-testing while she worked – whether or not she was hungry. And when she got home, she'd sit down to a traditional meal with her family.

Constantly being around food proved disastrous for Robin. By 1998, she was just shy of 21 stone. And she was miserable.

Robin knew enough about nutrition to realise that she was not eating out of need. She was eating out of habit. A habit fed by being around tasty, delicious food all day. She had completely lost touch with her internal hunger cues.

Robin's weight-loss strategy turned out to be one simple promise that she made to herself. "I told myself that I would eat only when I was hungry and that I would stop when I was satisfied – not stuffed, just satisfied," she explains. This forced her to listen to her body and think about why she wanted to eat *before* she put food in her mouth. "If I realised that I wasn't truly hungry, I'd distract myself until the impulse passed – usually by thinking about the pounds I'd gain if I gave in," she says.

By adjusting her eating pattern and making healthier food choices, Robin was able to take off 102 pounds in about a year. She's still working to reach her goal weight of 10st 9lb. Her conviction to lose weight is stronger than any urge to eat. "I felt an overwhelming desire to overeat only once," she notes. "Reminding myself of my goal and focusing on my success so far is what keeps me on track."

WINNING ACTION ➤ ➤ ➤

Listen to your body. Like Robin, I've learned to distinguish between when I'm actually hungry and when I'm just responding to the sight of tempting foods. It has made a huge difference in helping me keep my weight under control. Here's a trick that I find helpful. Before eating anything, ask yourself, "Am I really hungry?" Rate your hunger on a scale of zero to five (zero being the least hungry, five being the most). Let your body tell you how much to eat.

"SKINNY FOODS" CURE
A 50-YEAR WEIGHT PROBLEM

Helen Stein *loves* to eat. These days, the 73 year old eats more than ever – and she hasn't gained back an ounce of the 38 pounds that she lost 15 years ago.

How? By choosing foods that fill her up, not out.

Helen's battle of the bulge began 65 years ago, when she was just 8 years old. At the time, she turned to food to help ease the pain of her mother's death. That led to an unhealthy pattern of using food for comfort – and putting on pounds. She reached 12st 12lb during her first year at college and remained at that weight for years.

Even though she was heavier than she should have been, Helen didn't worry about it. She never liked the idea of dieting. The prospect of giving up her favourite foods and eating less repeatedly dissuaded her from slimming down.

Then, one morning, everything changed. "When I woke up, I said to myself, 'I'm tired of this,'" Helen recalls. "I didn't want to be heavy anymore. I wanted to be thin."

Looking back, Helen realises that her decision to lose weight had been brewing for some time. "I had grown unhappy with my appearance and, deep down, I wanted to be thin," she says. "The time had come to do something about it and I knew it."

As she planned her weight-loss strategy, Helen admitted to herself that she would have a hard time changing her diet. So instead of trying to eat less, she ate differently. She sought out foods that would leave her feeling full without supplying a lot of fat or calories. Most of Helen's lunches and dinners started out with a great big salad flavoured with balsamic vinegar. She thought nothing of snacking on a big pink grapefruit, a whole cantaloupe melon or a chunk of watermelon. She cooked with plenty of onions, oregano and other herbs to increase the satiety of her meals. "I discovered that the right seasonings could make low-fat foods quite satisfying," she says.

These simple changes allowed Helen to lose what she called her extra baggage in about 6 months. These days, she eats whenever she wants to, without worrying about her weight. She just makes sure to choose "skinny" foods that satisfy.

WINNING ACTION ➤ ➤ ➤

Fill up on fibre-rich foods. Helen's strategy of eating filling low-fat, low-calorie, high-fibre foods is smart for two reasons. First, fibre helps absorb fat calories and eliminate them from your body before they end up on your belly or thighs. In fact, 1 gram of fibre can absorb 7 calories of fat. Second, fibre fills you up. Avoiding feelings of deprivation is critical to adopting permanent dietary changes.

SHE'S A NATURAL AT WEIGHT LOSS

Carla Tuckerton lost and regained the same 15 to 20 pounds for about 15 years. She finally unloaded them for good after discovering natural foods.

Carla, a 44-year-old consultant, never seemed to have a problem losing weight when she wanted to. "I just kept close tabs on the number of calories that I consumed and when I reached my goal weight, I resumed my normal eating habits," she explains.

Of course, normal for Carla meant lots of ice cream, chocolate and high-fat frozen foods. Given her love of junk food, even she wasn't terribly surprised when the pounds returned. "My weight fluctuated between 8st 13lb and 10st 5lb for years," she says.

Then, during one of her self-styled diets, Carla noticed that she wasn't feeling especially well. She got a lot of headaches and she felt tired, nervous and irritable. "When I started thinking about it, I realised that I always felt that way when I was dieting," she says.

Suspicious that some food was causing her symptoms, Carla grabbed a pen and paper and wrote down everything that she had eaten in the previous 3 to 4 days. "When I looked over my list, I was appalled," she recalls. "Almost everything on it contained artificial sweeteners or loads of salt or was terribly processed. I was practically living on frozen dinners, low-calorie fizzy drinks and sugar-free jelly. No wonder I felt so lousy."

On the spot, Carla swore off anything that contained artificial ingredients or was overly processed. She made time to cook her own meals. She bought her fish and chicken from a farmers' market near her home and shopped for fruits and vegetables labelled "organically grown". Discouraged by the number of additives in many commercially prepared baked goods, she began making her own breads, rolls and muffins. Spring water replaced colas and she drank her tea unsweetened.

The changes paid off almost right away. "I felt better than I had in a long time," Carla says. And there was another, unexpected benefit: "I don't know why, but I seemed to lose weight more easily after switching to natural foods," she adds.

Sure enough, in less than 6 months, Carla managed to get rid of the extra weight that she had been carrying around for years. Her weight dropped to 8st 13lb – and stayed there.

Five years later, Carla hasn't gained back an ounce, a feat that she attributes to her commitment to natural foods. "I feel that I'm a much healthier person now than I was back then," she says. "I've been able to keep my weight where it belongs by eating foods that are naturally nutritious and good for me, instead of relying on foods made with artificial ingredients that make me sick. I feel great."

WINNING ACTION ➤ ➤ ➤

Try a natural approach to weight loss. *There's no scientific proof that switching from highly processed, additive-laden foods to fresh, natural foods can help you lose weight faster. Still, Carla may be on to something. Research has shown that people tend to overindulge in low-fat and fat-free processed foods. The trouble is that even though these foods have little or no fat, they are loaded with calories. On the other hand, fresh foods such as fruits, vegetables and whole grains are naturally low in fat as well as calories. You can eat more of them without worrying about weight gain. Besides, going natural may make you feel better and healthier – and may even help you live longer!*

THE FINE PRINT
PARED HER FIGURE

When you want to lose weight, how much you eat is just as important as what you eat. Phyllis Barbour found that out the hard way.

In 1993, Phyllis went on a special low-fat, low-salt diet after undergoing heart bypass surgery. She followed the diet to the letter. To her pleasant surprise, her weight dropped from 9st 4lb to 8st 2lb in about 3 months and stayed there for several years.

So she was understandably puzzled when, in 1997, her clothes started feeling a little snug. She was cooking and eating all the right foods and she worked out three or four times a week at a local health club. Plus, her job as a department store saleswoman kept her on her feet constantly.

"I was doing all the right things, yet I was still gaining weight," she says. "I couldn't figure out why."

Then one day, while eating a bagel, Phyllis picked up the package and read the nutrition label. She discovered that one of those big, doughy delectables equalled four servings of bread. "I was shocked," she says. "I had always counted it as just one serving."

That incident prompted Phyllis to check out the labels of some other foods that she ate regularly. She found more of the same: what she considered one serving was actually two or three – sometimes more.

"It became clear why I was gaining weight," Phyllis says. "I started paying closer attention to my serving sizes, even measuring portions when I needed to. It made a big difference almost immediately. My weight dropped back down to where it belonged."

Now aged 70, Phyllis remains vigilant about her serving sizes. And it shows: her weight is once again holding steady at 8st 2lb. "I'm glad that I figured out why I was gaining," she says. "I worked hard to slim down and I wasn't about to let all that effort go to waste."

WINNING ACTION ➤ ➤ ➤

Read those labels! Even low-fat and fat-free foods can cause you to gain weight if you eat too much of them. What they lack in fat they more than make up for in calories. So pay attention to the labels on packaged and processed foods.

HE LOST WEIGHT THE ASIAN WAY

In 1997, at the age of 38, Lenny Vargas discovered a harsh reality of parenting: 5- and 6-year-olds are tough to keep up with. At 17st 7lb, Lenny was left huffing and puffing while his two kids were off and running down the street.

Vowing to improve his physical fitness, Lenny started walking and doing calisthenics – situps, pushups, squats, toe touches and leg raises. He did only a few repetitions of each exercise at first, then gradually increased the number of reps over time. Although he didn't really lose pounds, he noticed a change in his fitness.

Still determined to lose weight, he decided to give up snacks and junk food for Lent. Voilà – the combination of smarter eating and regular exercise helped him slim down. He dropped 10 pounds in 2 months.

Then came a business trip to Thailand and other destinations in the Far East, where he fell in love with the food. The fresh vegetables, fish and rice were like none he had ever tasted. "I always liked fish and vegetables, but I really enjoyed the way they were prepared in some of the places I visited," says Lenny. Spicy-hot Thai dishes were especially memorable. "I could eat like this more often," he thought.

Back home, he was surprised to find that he hadn't gained an ounce on his trip. He figured he was on to something and enlisted the help of his wife, Kathy. They got some cookbooks and began experimenting with Asian cooking at home. Imagine their delight when they discovered that the diet they were adopting was credited with keeping Asians so healthy and trim!

Over the next 18 months, Lenny managed to take off another 50 pounds – a feat that he attributes to his continued commitment to exercise and his penchant for Asian cuisine. He has maintained his weight at 13st 3lb ever since. "My wife didn't have a weight problem – even after two kids – but she has held steady, too," he adds.

Thanks to his healthier lifestyle, Lenny is able to hold his own when playing with his kids. He has even taken up running. "Not too long ago, I had to get a physical for my job," he says. "The doctor told me that my cholesterol, blood pressure and other vital signs were all at healthy levels for a man my age." Even though he isn't jetting off to Asia as frequently anymore, Lenny hasn't forgotten the valuable lessons from the Far East.

HE SHOPPED HIMSELF SLIMMER

Pete Falk never sets foot in a food shop without a plan – a menu plan, that is. Writing down exactly what he needs to prepare each week's meals keeps him away from all of the high-fat, high-calorie temptations that line supermarket aisles. It's the key to how he lost 63 pounds.

Pete, a 35-year-old computer engineer, got in the menu-plan habit while attending a medical clinic specialising in weight loss. At the time, he weighed 18st 5lb, too much even for his 6-foot-1-inch frame. "I had been heavy since I was a kid," he explains. "I wanted to slim down and I had tried numerous times on my own. I didn't get really motivated until my allergies and asthma started getting worse. Then I knew that I needed help."

At the clinic, Pete went on a medically-supervised eating plan for the first couple of months. Then, he worked with the doctor and a nutritionist, learning how to make smart food choices on his own. "They gave me sample menus, which I took to the supermarket with me so I'd know what to buy," he says. "Eventually, I realised that by sticking with the menus, I was filling my cart with healthy foods, not the junk that helped me gain in the first place."

The menus encouraged Pete to make other healthy changes

in his eating habits. He stopped skipping breakfast, he started packing his lunch on workdays and he tried to have dinner at about the same time every evening. "Because of my job, I had been eating really late some nights – around 10 o'clock," he says. "I was so hungry by then that I'd stuff myself."

As Pete's eating habits improved, his waistline shrank. He joined a local gym, where he worked out 6 days a week. Within 4 months he was 63 pounds lighter.

That was more than 2 years ago. Pete has since started lifting weights, which has added some bulk – all muscle – to his physique. He's holding steady at a fit 14st 4lb.

While exercising regularly has helped Pete get in shape, eating healthily has kept him trim. These days, he writes his own menus, but he still takes them to the shops. "My menus help me shop conscientiously," he says. "I get the right ingredients and buy only what I need – no junk food."

WINNING ACTION ➤ ➤ ➤

Get a plan. If you're prone to straying down the wrong supermarket aisle, like Pete, get a plan. Decide on your meals for a full week. Write down what you need to make each meal. Use that as your shopping list. This way, you'll leave the supermarket with exactly what you went in for and you'll minimise impulse buys.

SHE SHED HER SWEET TOOTH AND LOST 60 POUNDS

Maye Musk was the victim of an out-of-control sweet tooth. But once she declared her home a treat-free zone, she was able to lose 60 pounds.

For years, Maye had struggled with a seemingly insatiable

appetite. "Once I started eating, I couldn't stop," says the model and registered dietitian. "I didn't get full very easily." And her greatest weaknesses were sweets, biscuits, doughnuts and cakes.

Maye became a model at the age of 16. As her weight crept upwards to 14st 4lb, she moved into plus-size modelling and remained as popular as ever. But she was also becoming more self-conscious about her appearance.

Then one day while Maye was driving, her daughter reached over and jiggled the flab under her arms. "She thought it looked funny," Maye recalls. "I said to myself, 'I'm sick and tired of wearing jackets to hide my body, of wearing clothes without a waist, of not being able to tuck a shirt into jeans.'"

At that moment, Maye made up her mind: she was going to slim down and she would do whatever was necessary to accomplish her goal.

Her first task was to tame her penchant for sweet foods. She knew that if she didn't bring those goodies home, she wouldn't eat them. So she stopped buying them.

Then, she filled her refrigerator and cupboards with healthy, low-fat foods, such as fruits and vegetables, yogurt and rice cakes. And she began exercising – walking, riding an exercise bike, practising yoga.

By eating better and working out, Maye was able to lose most of her extra weight within 8 months. "It took another 6 months for the last 15 pounds to go," she says. That was 10 years ago.

These days, you won't find a single sweet or biscuit in Maye's apartment. Nor will you find Maye fretting over her figure. At the age of 51, she usually carries a healthy 10 stone on her 5-foot-8-inch frame. She continues to model part-time. And she uses her training as a dietitian and her personal experience in slimming down to speak on weight loss, healthy eating, body image, appearance and self-esteem.

SHE LOST 100 POUNDS IN THE FRUIT AND VEG AISLE

After the birth of her second daughter, Melissa Katz was stunned to discover that her weight had settled in at 17st 2lb. The veteran yo-yo dieter found herself at a crossroads.

"I thought, 'If I don't get a handle on this now, I'm going to be fat my whole life,'" she says.

She decided to join Weight Watchers. After a few meetings, she realised just how much food she had been eating each and every day. "No wonder I had gained so much weight," she says. "The problem was that I was used to eating big meals and big snacks. I felt hungry all the time."

Weight Watchers taught her that she could have plenty of food – if she made the right choices. So she turned to fruits and vegetables to fill her plate. "They made me feel full without supplying lots of calories," she explains.

As the weight started to melt away, her self-esteem grew. "As I became more confident, I became more physically active," she says.

It took only a year for Melissa to lose 100 pounds. She has maintained that loss for 2½ years. And her casual interest in exercise has turned into a career as a physical trainer.

But what Melissa, aged 35, is most proud of is the impact that her new eating habits are having on her daughters. "They make good food choices, too," she says. "They'll pick a piece of fruit over a piece of cake. That's what gives me the biggest joy."

BREAKFAST MADE HER
A WEIGHT-LOSS CHAMPION

For years, Susan Carlson couldn't stomach the thought of eating in the morning. But only after becoming a breakfast loyalist did she lose 36 pounds.

Faced with choosing between a bowl of cereal and another 15 minutes of sleep, Susan would always go for the extra snooze time. "Food first thing in the morning never appealed to me," says the 42-year-old sales manager.

Because she would eat dinner at around 6:00 p.m. and then skip breakfast, Susan was going foodless for up to 18 hours at a stretch. By noon, she'd be famished. So she'd plunge into a huge lunch, then spend the rest of the day snacking on biscuits and crisps.

By the time Susan reached her early thirties, she weighed 12st 13lb. She was so embarrassed about her appearance that she stopped going to clothes shops. "I only ordered out of catalogues – always clothing with elastic waists," she recalls.

After several unsuccessful weight-loss attempts, Susan asked some of her slender friends how they stay slim. Their answer: breakfast. Susan started slowly, with one slice of toast and a cup of coffee. She eventually added a bowl of cereal or porridge to her morning meal. To her surprise, she was less hungry at lunch and her midday munching stopped.

Now, her favourite breakfast foods include porridge, cereal with strawberries and wholemeal toast with a slice of cheese. Susan lost 36 pounds in less than a year. Her slimmer figure has made her a breakfast believer.

> ## WINNING ACTION ➤➤➤
>
> *Eat a real breakfast. Many women, like Susan, skip breakfast – and overeat all day as a result. Research shows that people who eat a healthy and hearty breakfast are thinner than those who eat no breakfast at all. That's because breakfast helps boost your metabolism, so you burn calories more efficiently all day. For years, I skipped breakfast, too. Now, I make sure to grab something in the morning: a banana, a cereal bar or some yogurt. It's amazing how much more energy I have until lunchtime.*

HIS KITCHEN CLOSES AT 8 O' CLOCK

When Dave Venne moved in with some of his friends, he was looking forward to the companionship and fun. What he didn't expect was a 15-pound weight gain.

"Those guys ate all the time and I was right there with them," says the 25-year-old landscaping-design supervisor. "Still, I couldn't believe how quickly the pounds piled up. I went from 16st 1lb to 17st 2lb in 12 weeks. More than a pound a week!"

At 6 foot 4 inches, Dave carried the extra weight well. But it made him feel heavy and uncomfortable. "I work outside in the heat and I felt miserable," he says. "Plus, I wasn't running as fast or jumping as high when I played basketball, one of my favourite pastimes.

"My flatmates and I would play basketball or do something else for a couple of hours practically every night," he continues.

"By the time we finished, we'd be so hungry that we'd eat just about anything that we could get our hands on." Their foods of choice were pizza, burgers and Chinese takeaway, all washed down with copious quantities of fizzy drinks and beer. "Sometimes, I'd eat an entire pizza and drink three or four beers, plus a couple of Cokes, before going to bed," Dave says. "And that was on top of eating a sandwich or something else when I got home from work."

Feeling out of shape and overweight, Dave decided his late-night eating habits had to go. "I figured that if I ate a good dinner, I wouldn't get hungry later that night," he says. "I'm not much of a cook, but even I can heat up a can of soup and put together a turkey sandwich."

As he began paying more attention to his food choices, his other meals became healthier, too. He traded in his usual sausage-egg-and-cheese breakfast sandwich for a bowl of cereal, a glass of orange juice and sometimes toast. For lunch, he still favoured fast-food restaurants, but he replaced his bacon double cheese-burgers with grilled chicken sandwiches. And he carried bottles of water with him everywhere. "I have to drink a lot while I'm working," he explains. "I used to down seven or eight fizzy drinks a day. I think that switching to water helped me lose weight."

Indeed, Dave got rid of those 15 extra pounds, plus 8 more, in about 6 months. He has held steady at 15st 7lb, a comfortable weight for his size, since 1998.

These days, Dave seldom eats after 8 o'clock at night. If he feels hungry after a couple of hours of shooting hoops, he'll eat fruit or fat-free frozen yogurt. When his flatmates order takeaway, he helps himself to a healthy snack or goes to bed instead.

"Being around junk food and not eating any of it was hard at first," Dave admits. "But now I feel so much better about myself that I don't even miss that stuff."

WINNING ACTION ➤ ➤ ➤

For dinner, be an early bird. Dave is doing the right thing by putting a lid on his late-night noshing. Research has shown that the later you eat, the more likely it is that your body will store the food as fat. So try to eat your last meal or snack of the day before 8:00 p.m. If you get hungry late at night, choose a low-fat, high-volume food such as unsugared popcorn or an apple.

LENTEN PROMISE LED TO 20-POUND REWARD

If you're having a hard time pinpointing the hidden calories in your diet, take a tip from Jim Gorman. The 33-year-old public relations supervisor will tell you to look in the bottom of your empty glass. He knows from experience.

In 1995, Jim gave up all sugary beverages and alcohol for Lent, resolving to drink only water and soda water. By the time Easter rolled around, he was 20 pounds lighter. "I wasn't really looking to lose weight," he says. "But I have to admit that I was a bit bulkier than I wanted to be."

Since then, Jim has kept his weight between 11st 4lb and 11st 9lb, appropriate for his 5-foot-11-inch frame. He attributes his trim physique to his continued ban on sugary beverages. "Staying away from fizzy drinks, sweetened iced tea and other flavoured drinks has made all the difference on the scales," he says.

While Jim sticks with water at home, he may order a beer or two when he's socialising with friends. "I don't worry too much about the calories from an occasional brew," he explains. "After all, 90 per cent of the time I'm drinking only water and that has no calories."

SHE'S ONE SMART COOKIE

Lesli Hicks used to think that a meal just wasn't complete unless it ended with a sweet – until she faced going to her 10-year school reunion 35 pounds heavier.

A steady diet of chocolate, cakes, biscuits and pastries transformed Lesli from trim to tubby. Once a slim 7st 7lb in school, she was pushing 10 stone a decade later when the invitation to her class reunion arrived. "I wasn't obese, but I definitely weighed a lot more than I should have," she says. "I didn't want my old classmates to see how much I had gained."

Determination set in. Out went the cakes, doughnuts and other confections that had become part of Lesli's mealtime routine. "I knew that I couldn't eat just a little dessert," she says. "It was either all or nothing." To satisfy her sweet tooth, she concluded her meals with natural sweets – primarily apples, pears and other fruits.

Lesli's discipline paid off. Within a few weeks, she whittled 10 pounds from her 5-foot-2½-inch frame. She went to her class reunion feeling fit and fantastic. "I looked better than ever – even better than when I was seven and a half stone," she says.

After the reunion, Lesli lost even more weight. Within a few weeks, she was down to 8st 10lb, where she has stayed ever since. Now aged 37, she'd like to take off several more pounds to reach 8st 3 or 4lb. She sticks with her weight-loss regime by allowing herself one dessert splurge a week. "When I'm tempted for more, I ask myself, 'Am I going to feel better or worse after I eat that?'" she says. "Usually, I tell myself that I'll feel worse and I pass up the food."

WINNING ACTION ➤ ➤ ➤

Indulge in dessert – but only when you really need it. Cheesecake, hot-fudge sundaes and other high-fat goodies have their place in a healthy diet, as long as they're not everyday fare. At other times, you can satisfy your sweet tooth with low-fat treats. Besides fresh fruit, there's angel food cake (0.1 gram of fat per serving), fig rolls (1 gram), fortune cookies (0 gram) and rice pudding (4 grams).

AN ORANGE LED HER TO SWEET SUCCESS

It wasn't until Susan Ledford discovered the power of a fresh, sweet orange that she was able to pass up her biggest indulgence and lose 43 pounds.

A member of a big family that loves food, Susan is no stranger to temptation. When special occasions call for family celebrations, "it's like a race to see who can make the most disgustingly rich casserole," says the 36-year-old newspaper designer.

Such decadent dishes were standard fare while Susan was growing up. But they weren't kind to her waistline. She gained weight throughout her teenage years and by her twenties, she was trying all sorts of diets in an effort to slim down. "I'd go on one diet and lose a few pounds only to watch them return when I went back to my normal eating habits," she recalls. By 34, she topped out at 12 stone.

Knowing that Susan was unhappy with her figure, a friend suggested that she join Weight Watchers. The programme taught Susan how to make healthy food choices and control her portion sizes. Within a year, she took off 43 pounds.

Thrilled to have finally reached her goal weight of 8st 13lb, Susan was determined to stay there. But she had one dietary hurdle to overcome. Susan loved to bake biscuits for her family and friends, especially around the Christmas holidays. She especially enjoyed licking the bowl and sampling each batch fresh from the oven.

Realising that her taste-testing ways would do nothing for her hard-earned figure, Susan decided to have a healthy snack before baking. Her food of choice: a fresh, juicy orange. She found that the intense flavour of the fruit quashed her cravings for biscuits. She was able to bake to her heart's content without eating a thing.

Thanks to her ingenious strategy, Susan had an easier time sticking with her healthy eating habits. Her weight has held steady at 8st 13lb since 1998.

WINNING ACTION ➤ ➤ ➤

Feed your sweet tooth an orange. Susan's strategy has real scientific merit. According to Marilyn C. Majchrzak, R.D., food-development manager at the Canyon Ranch Spa/Health Resort in Tucson, Arizona, intensely flavoured foods such as oranges tend to be more satisfying than bland foods. So snacking on something sweet and juicy will help reduce temptation. Keep lots of oranges, fresh pineapple, strawberries or your favourite tastebud-shocking fruit in your fridge.

A BRUSH STROKE OF GENIUS

Ask Lisa Gardiner about her favourite weight-loss weapon and she's likely to show you her toothbrush. After all, it helped her take off 25 pounds in just 6 months.

After two pregnancies, Lisa was eager to slim down. But caring for her newborn twin daughters and 3-year-old son didn't leave her much time to plan nutritious meals or stick with an exercise routine. Lisa believed that if she could control her after-dinner noshing, she'd take a significant bite out of her fat and calorie intake. So she used a little trick that she had used to lose 20 pounds in college.

Instead of heading to the kitchen right after dinner, Lisa would head to the bathroom and brush her teeth. "It was my signal that my time to eat was over for the day," she says. "If I felt the urge to snack, I just reminded myself that I had already brushed my teeth."

This simple strategy helped Lisa, aged 35, slim down for the second – and, she's determined – last time in her life.

WINNING ACTION ➤ ➤ ➤

Try the toothbrush trick. After dinner, brush your teeth. This simple task sends a message to your brain that you've finished eating for the day. What's more, the toothpaste alters the flavour of food. If you were to eat something after brushing, it wouldn't taste very good. What's more, your teeth and your smile will thank you!

SHE STUCK TO HER DIET WITH CHEWING GUM

For Ann Marie Grathwol, losing weight and keeping it off was just a matter of keeping her mouth occupied.

Weary of hauling around an extra 35 pounds, Ann Marie plunged into an exercise programme at her local gym, became a vegetarian and swore off fried foods. The changes were dramatic – and successful: after several months, she dropped four dress sizes.

But like many, the 32 year old liked to snack, particularly on chocolate. She often munched when she was under stress or bored. "It wasn't that I was really hungry," she says. "My mouth was just looking for something to do."

Ann Marie worried that she would put back on the weight she had worked so hard to lose. Then, by accident, she discovered the appetite-suppressing magic of sugarless gum. By chewing gum, Ann Marie found that she was able to stay away from chocolate and other high-fat goodies. "The sweet, minty flavour and the chewing made me much less likely to snack," she says. "It provided the tension relief that I was looking for in food."

Her snack cravings under control, Ann Marie kept off the weight. And now, whenever she finds herself having a snack attack, she simply pulls out a stick of gum and chews.

WINNING ACTION ➤➤➤

Keep your mouth occupied. Chewing gum can help distract you from the urge to snack. Like Ann Marie, take advantage of peppermint's appetite-suppressant qualities for more weight-loss power. Whatever flavour you choose, make sure it's sugarless – it's kinder to your teeth.

MILK STOPPED HER FROM SNACKING

Janet Parent knew that to lose weight, she needed to gain control of her eating habits. She did it with milk.

Janet grew up in a family whose clean-your-plate philosophy was largely responsible for her eventual size-16 figure. Over the years, she dieted time and again, sometimes shedding a few pounds. But she'd lie awake at night, feeling starved. Inevitably, she'd return to large meals and constant snacking.

Over a lifetime of gaining, losing and regaining, Janet watched herself hit a high of 11st 10lb. Finally, at the age of 64, she became determined to slim down. "It was either buy yet another new wardrobe or take off the weight," she says.

Her first step was to drop her drastic dieting and go back to preparing and eating her regular foods. For Janet, that meant meals of steak, potatoes and sweetcorn; or chicken, rice and broccoli – both always served with a salad. The main difference was that she began to leave a little food on her plate at the end of every meal.

This trick helped Janet control her portion sizes. But she still craved snacks. So she tried drinking skimmed milk between meals as a way to take the edge off her hunger. "I like the taste of milk and I knew from experience that drinking it made me feel full," she explains. "Besides, the extra calcium is good for my bones." She also ate an orange every night before going to bed, to keep her stomach full until morning and stave off the midnight munchies. Slowly but surely, the extra pounds came off – and have stayed off for 2 years.

Today, at the age of 66, Janet weighs 10st 7lb and wears a size-12 dress. "Drinking milk is the easiest thing I've ever done to lose weight," she says.

WINNING ACTION ▶ ▶ ▶

Satisfy your hunger with skimmed milk. A cold 8-fl oz (240-ml) glass of skimmed milk is not only filling but also healthy – a great source of bone-building calcium. If you aren't a fan of skimmed milk, try semi-skimmed. It has a richer taste but each serving still gets fewer than 30 per cent of its calories from fat. If you're a chocoholic, add 2 tablespoons of low-sugar chocolate syrup for a fast chocolate fix.

LOSE WHILE YOU SNOOZE

When nighttime noshing threatened to derail Cheryl Lachenmayer's weight-loss efforts, she didn't give in. Instead, she turned in – and lost 40 pounds.

For most of her adult life, Cheryl maintained a healthy weight without any type of dieting. But that changed after the birth of her two daughters. A 50-pound gain during each pregnancy catapulted her out of her normal weight range. At 12st 2lb, Cheryl was on the verge of qualifying as clinically obese.

She joined Weight Watchers. She knew that the organisation's low-fat meal plan would provide a structure for developing healthy new eating habits.

But new habits take time to form. And during those first weeks, Cheryl faced the same dilemma every day. She had no problem sticking with her meal plan at breakfast and lunch. But staying on track through dinner required more effort. By evening, her resolve crumbled. She'd get intense cravings – often for ice cream or cheese and crackers.

Cheryl's solution? When her willpower quit for the day, so did she. Rather than cave in to cravings, she simply went to bed. Sometimes, as early as 9 o'clock. She felt a little silly going to bed so early, but it worked. Cheryl lost 40 pounds over 7 to 8 months.

WINNING ACTION ➤ ➤ ➤

Get a good night's sleep. According to a study at Case Western Reserve University in Cleveland, there is a limit to the amount of willpower that a person can exert in a single day. That limit is highly individual. But as a general rule, when you start to hear the call of nighttime cravings, that can be your cue to turn in for the evening. You can sleep off your cravings and wake up with rejuvenated resolve.

SHE'S SLIMMER – AND SO ARE HER FAVOURITE RECIPES

Teresa Tomeo grew up in a traditional Italian family that loves traditional Italian meals. Huge plates of spaghetti, bowls of meatballs and thickly buttered bread are staples at family gatherings. And it shows: many of Teresa's relatives are overweight.

But not Teresa – not anymore. Her secret? She learned to make slimmer versions of her favourite Italian dishes.

Teresa's weight-loss odyssey began in 1985. Then aged 25 and a successful radio news reporter, she was trying hard to break into television news, with no success. Finally, a friend laid it on the line: at 13st 8lb, Teresa was too fat for TV.

The remark stung, but Teresa knew that her friend was right. She wasn't about to let her weight stop her from realising her career goals. So she enrolled in a medically supervised weight-loss programme that included a written eating plan and weekly weigh-ins. Within 7 months, she lost 60 pounds.

Teresa was thrilled with her new, trim figure and she vowed not to let those pounds come back. So, armed with the nutrition knowledge that she had gleaned from her weight-loss programme, she began experimenting with her favourite Italian recipes, looking for ways to lighten them. She reduced the amount of olive oil in her tomato sauce to just a drizzle. And she took out the meat completely, replacing it with vegetables. She used vegetable purées to thicken sauces as well as soups. She topped salads with a squeeze of lemon.

By turning her kitchen into a laboratory and reinventing her recipe collection, Teresa has managed to maintain her weight at a healthy 9st 4lb for 14 years. Along the way, she realised her dream of working in television news, landing a job with a TV station. She stayed there for 10 years before returning to radio, which she calls her real love, in 1998.

SHE HELD THE MAYO AND LOST 15 POUNDS

Little things mean a lot, especially when it comes to weight loss. Just ask Barbara Rodriguez.

The 23 year old had never been seriously overweight, "just a bit chunky," she says. But when she got engaged in 1997, she decided that she wanted to look just right for her wedding. That meant slimming down – the right way. "I didn't want to fall for any of those fad diets," she recalls.

Barbara began reading books on nutrition and weight. She soon realised that certain seemingly innocuous foods such as mayonnaise, butter, cheese, salad dressing and sour cream were adding a boatload of fat and calories to her meals. So she dropped them.

Now, instead of putting sour cream on her baked potato, she sprinkles a little salt. She flavours her salads with vinegar rather than dressing, her sandwiches with mustard rather than mayonnaise. And she bulks up her sandwiches with lettuce and tomato, not cheese.

Since she started making her simple substitutions, Barbara has lost and kept off 15 pounds. And she doesn't even miss her high-fat, high-calorie flavour enhancers. "I would never deprive myself of my favourite foods," she adds. "I just eat them in moderation."

Best of all, she no longer considers herself chunky. Losing those 15 pounds put her in a slim size-8 wedding dress.

WINNING ACTION ➤ ➤ ➤

Flavour your foods with calorie burners. Like Barbara, you can whittle away at your fat and calorie intakes just by replacing high-fat, high-calorie condiments with healthier alternatives. In fact, certain spicy condiments such as horseradish and chilli powder actually speed your body's metabolic rate, so you burn more calories. Try mixing a small amount of chilli powder, cumin, chopped cucumbers and green onions into low-fat crème fraîche or yogurt. Use this calorie-burning Mexican topping to flavour grilled chicken breasts or on a jacket potato.

SHE SWITCHED PLATES AND LOST 5 STONE

Toni Willis lost five dress sizes. All she had to do was change the way that she sets her table.

At 15st 5lb and eager to slim down, Toni finally got fed up with fad diets that didn't work. She decided to put into practice some advice that she had received from a nutritionist a few years before, during her pregnancy. "I didn't tell anyone about my plan because I didn't want people reminding me about it all the time," she says. "I just woke up one morning and said, 'Today's the day.'"

Out went the eggs, bacon, sausage, burgers, chips and *anything* with cheese. In their place were muffins with peanut butter, bagels, baked fish, chicken, pasta and plenty of fruits and vegetables.

To help control the amount of food that she ate, Toni applied that old adage "out of sight, out of mind" to her dinner table. When preparing meals for herself and her family, she stopped serving family style. Instead, she divvied up all of the food among five plates, one for each family member. For herself, she used a salad plate, so it looked full even with smaller portions. As soon as she had finished eating, she got up and left the room. That way, she wasn't tempted to nibble.

Toni adjusted to her new eating habits surprisingly easily. And once she started losing weight, she didn't struggle with her food choices or portion sizes. In fact, she learned to love the healthier foods.

"I was so into losing weight that I didn't overeat. If anything, there were times when I didn't eat enough," she says. "To me, there was no food that was worth the calories."

Today, at 36, Toni is 5 stone lighter. She has maintained a healthy weight of 10st 5lb for 2 years. She says that she eats just the right amount of food and she doesn't go back for seconds and thirds. "I never feel like I'm depriving myself of anything," she says. "Sometimes, I just have a bite of something decadent and toss the rest. I never feel stuffed."

WINNING ACTION ➤ ➤ ➤

Pick your perfect plate. This is a great tip – and with a husband who is 6 foot 4 inches and a huge eater, I follow it religiously. Instead of using a regular dinner plate for my main meal, I substitute a salad plate or dessert plate. It's an easy way to control portion sizes. In fact, a salad plate holds only about 60 per cent of the food that fits on a dinner plate. And the full plate serves as a visual cue for my brain: it thinks that I'm getting a lot of food, so I feel satisfied with less.

SHE STOPPED "CLEANING UP" AND LOST THE LAST 10

For Sharon Poppendeck, having her second child at the age of 39 was a welcome joy. But the post-pregnancy pounds that lingered a year later were just plain unwelcome.

Sharon had read that metabolism starts to slow at around the age of 40. But she couldn't understand why the extra 10 pounds that had accumulated around her belly and thighs just wouldn't go away, no matter how hard she tried to shed it.

Puzzled, she began scrutinising her eating habits like a scientist searching for a new discovery. Healthy foods? Yes. Snacks? No. She didn't even eat when she took the kids for their favourite fast-food meals. Or did she?

Sharon didn't usually order, but she did eat – everything the kids didn't. "I'd just pick it up and finish it so I didn't have to throw it out," she says. "I didn't even notice that I was doing it."

Now, when she takes the kids out for fast food, she eats her typical healthy meal beforehand so that she's not tempted to finish their leftovers. And forget the guilt about throwing away food. Into the rubbish bin it goes!

Sharon also made another discovery and adopted a no-eating policy in her car. "I would always carry little snacks with me in case the kids got hungry," she says. "The problem was that every time I gave them a handful of crackers, I ate a handful, too!" She still carries snacks for her children, but she herself doesn't eat them.

Sure enough, the weight came off. And Sharon, now 42, says that it has remained off, thanks to her bit of detective work.

WINNING ACTION ➤ ➤ ➤

Leave the leftovers. Unlike what you may have learned growing up, you are not a human waste disposal. So don't feel compelled to eat your kids' or grandkids' leftovers. If you can't bear to throw out uneaten food, wrap it up and put it in the refrigerator for later. In restaurants, request a doggie bag – unless you're going to be too tempted to eat the leftovers yourself. In that case, let the waiter take it away.

SHE SLIMMED DOWN BY SITTING DOWN

When it comes to eating, Kathy Wilson was a stand-up person. She would stand at the cupboard and snack. She would stand at the refrigerator and snack. "I can honestly say that I never sat down and ate a meal," says the 48 year old.

By the time she reached her mid-forties, Kathy weighed 18st 10lb. Her blood pressure was way above normal. And she no longer wanted to go out with her husband, because she was embarrassed by her size.

All of these factors drove Kathy to confront her weight problem. She knew that she had to slim down, but how?

After looking into several weight-loss programmes, Kathy decided to enroll with the US-based group, Jenny Craig. In the programme, clients eat prepackaged meals until they're halfway to their goal weights. Then they switch to preparing their own food, using menus provided by Jenny Craig. "Typically, when you think of a diet, you think of what you can't eat," Kathy says. "But I learned that I can eat what I want, as long as I control my portions."

She also learned to stop sabotaging her weight-loss programme by eating in front of the fridge. "When I started adding up the calories, I realised that I was taking in a lot more than I should have been, mostly because of my stand-up meals and snacks," Kathy says. "Sitting down at the kitchen or dining room table each time I ate forced me to be more aware of the food that I was putting in my mouth."

Within a year of starting the programme, Kathy had lost 100 pounds. She has maintained her goal weight of 11st 8lb since April 1994.

Now that she's slimmer, Kathy is more active than she used to be. She loves to run, ice-skate and play softball. She was so impressed with how the programme changed her life that she became the director of a Jenny Craig centre. "I want to help others achieve their weight-loss goals, as I have," she says.

WINNING ACTION ➤ ➤ ➤

Leave stand-up to the comedians. Research shows that nearly all of us, whether we're heavy or slim, underestimate by 20 to 50 per cent how much we eat. Like Kathy, we forget about the snacking in front of the refrigerator, the taste-testing during meal preparation, the nibbling during meetings at work. And those calories can add up fast. To keep tabs on absentminded eating, get in the habit of sitting at the table for every meal and snack. This simple action will help remind you that what you're putting in your mouth counts towards your daily calorie intake. You may realise that you're not as hungry as you thought!

WATER BECAME HER APPETISER

Maureen Pence lost 45 pounds by drowning her appetite before every meal.

Maureen had resigned herself to being overweight. She liked

to eat and dined out often. But when her father, a retired doctor, suffered a heart attack, her attitude changed. At 31, she knew that she had to get serious about slimming down. So she followed the standard weight-loss advice, trying to eat more healthily and exercise more. This was easy enough – when she was at home.

Maureen's job as a production manager for a chemical company required her to eat out frequently with clients. Finding something relatively healthy to order from the menu usually wasn't a problem. But the portions were huge and Maureen – well, she was hungry.

Then one day, Maureen drank a full glass of water before she went to a restaurant. She found she wasn't as ravenous when she ordered and she didn't wolf down her meal. In fact, she left some of her food uneaten. Quite by accident, she had discovered a weight-loss trick.

"I started drinking a big glass of water before all my meals and taking sips between bites," Maureen says. "I was amazed at how full it made me feel."

Gradually, she was able to lose 45 pounds. Today, at 36 and 10st 13lb, Maureen is a slender and happy size 12.

WINNING ACTION ➤ ➤ ➤

Start every meal with water. Like Maureen, you can keep your appetite in check by drinking an 8-fl oz (240-ml) glass of water before every meal. And make sure the water is ice cold; your body has to burn almost 8 calories to raise the water temperature to body temperature. In fact, if you were to drink eight 8-fl oz glasses of ice-cold water a day, you'd burn about 62 calories. That adds up to more than a pound's worth of calories in just 2 months.

SHE SLIMMED DOWN BY SCHEDULING HER SPLURGES

During the week, Helene Gullaksen is spartan about her food choices. But when the weekend arrives, she lets loose. "I eat whatever I please," says the 35 year old. "I shop for special treats, I go out for dinner with my husband and sometimes I pig out on pizza."

Relaxing her strict dietary rules on weekends keeps Helene from feeling deprived. It also helped her lose 50 pounds.

Like many women, Helene didn't have a weight problem until after her two pregnancies. "With my first baby, I went from 9st 6lb to 12st 12lb," she recalls. "I managed to lose about 38 pounds before I got pregnant again." After giving birth to her second child, she kept right on gaining, eventually reaching 13st 8lb.

As much as Helene wanted to unload the extra pounds, she recoiled at the thought of dieting. "I enjoy eating and I didn't want to feel deprived," she explains. So she made a deal with herself: if she ate healthily during the week, she could splurge on weekends.

Helene follows a weekday diet that's quite austere, limiting the number of calories that she consumes. Her typical breakfast consists of a whole-grain roll with olives and sun-dried tomatoes. For lunch, she chooses between a low-calorie frozen ready meal and a selection of buffet items from a restaurant near her workplace. "I don't even look at the 'bad' foods," she says. "I just fill my plate with beans, fresh vegetables and fresh fruits."

At dinnertime, she prepares a meal for her family, then serves herself half-portions of whatever they're having.

Helene still faces temptations during the week. But knowing that she can splurge on weekends gives her incentive to stay true to her weekday diet. "When I get a craving during the week, I tell myself, 'It's not the last time that I'll have an opportunity to eat this food,'" she says. "I can walk away from whatever is tempting me much more easily."

Helene's weekdays-on, weekends-off eating plan – and walking whenever she gets a chance – helped her go from 13st 8lb to 9st 9lb in just 9 months. She has maintained her weight since 1997.

As much as she enjoys her weekend respites, Helene says that her splurges are more low-key than they used to be. In fact, she no longer experiences cravings for sweets or ice cream, two of her former favourite foods. "I try to listen to my body and give it what it asks for, no more and no less," she says.

WINNING ACTION ➤ ➤ ➤

Take a weekend break. Weekends are made for rest and rejuvenation, so give yourself those 2 days to relax your dietary guidelines. Feel free to enjoy some of the foods that are off limits during the week, but don't go overboard. I have found that by designating Saturdays and Sundays as my moderate-splurge days, I have an easier time sticking with my healthy eating plan during the rest of the week.

HE HIT THE ROAD TO WEIGHT LOSS SUCCESS

Rob Christie credits a cool box with helping him lose 60 pounds.

A fortysomething entrepreneur, Rob had been thin for most of his life. That changed when he decided to start his own business. Soon, he was practically living in his car, driving from one sales call to the next. When he grabbed a bite to eat, it was usually at the nearest fast-food restaurant.

Five years and hundreds of cheeseburgers later, Rob was severely overweight and out of shape.

His low point came the day he found himself lying in bed, unable to move because of intense back pain. "I knew my lifestyle and the extra weight were contributing to the problem," he said. "Right then, I committed to getting my health back."

His first step was to make an appointment with a personal trainer. With the trainer's guidance, Rob began a regular fitness programme consisting of two 30-minute strength-training sessions each week. That prompted him to overhaul his eating habits.

That's when he bought a cool box.

Instead of stopping at fast-food joints and munching all day on whatever he found handy, Rob began stocking his cool box with healthy foods – usually a low-fat turkey sandwich or tuna sandwich for lunch, along with fresh fruits, raw vegetables, yogurt and a cereal bar.

Before hitting the road, he enjoyed a low-fat breakfast of porridge and fruit at home. At dinnertime, he ate a balanced meal consisting of lean meat, plenty of vegetables and a modest serving of pasta or another starch. All the while, he was continuing his twice-weekly workouts.

In just 6 months, Rob lost 60 pounds. One year later, he's a fit and muscular 14st 9lb. "Losing that weight and getting in shape has increased my energy level tremendously," Rob says. "I feel 25 instead of 45!"

WINNING ACTION ➤ ➤ ➤

Stock up for road trips. Rob's strategy really works. Whenever I'm travelling for business or pleasure I always make sure to put something healthy – a cereal bar, a banana or pretzels – in my briefcase or travel bag. I feel better knowing that I can eat nutritious low-fat foods and I get there more relaxed because I don't have to wait in long food queues.

SHE TRAVELS WITH HER LUNCH BAG

" 'We need you in San Francisco in 48 hours,' " shouts Rosanna Pittella, mimicking her job's frequent demands for air travel. "Usually, I'd travel light and come home with 10 extra pounds."

She's exaggerating, of course, but not by much. At one time, the 41-year-old consulting-firm director and mother of three carried 18st 11lb on her 5-foot-2-inch frame. She blames the excess baggage on the sheer exhaustion of making repeated long-distance trips. "When you're that tired, you eat what's convenient – and that often means unhealthy foods," she says. "And once I'd blow it, I'd feel sick the whole trip. It sets up a cycle of bad eating."

Finally, Rosanna wised up to her unhealthy ways. Temptation is greatest when you're out of your routine," she says. So, "I pack an emergency food kit, using an insulated lunch bag," she explains. "I fill it with cans of tuna, small cans of vegetables, canned snack packs of fruit that are for kids' lunches (the portion sizes are perfect), fresh fruit and bottled water. That way, I'm not a victim of airport food or late-night room service because it's the only thing available."

Today, a year later and 103 pounds lighter, Rosanna is happy, comfortable and soaring with energy. She says that packing her emergency food kit is like brushing her teeth. "I won't leave the house without doing either one," she says. "They're so much a part of me that I can't avoid them."

WINNING ACTION ➤ ➤ ➤

Flying? Don't forget your food. You don't have to be a frequent flier like Rosanna to face the nutritional pitfalls of air travel. Prepare for your hunger and pack healthy snacks in your hand luggage. Take some water, too. Aeroplane cabins are extremely dehydrating.

SHE GETS HALF
OF HER MEAL TO GO

After years of frustration, Mary Ellen O'Grady finally found a weight-loss device that works for her: the venerable doggie bag.

At 37, she noticed that even though her eating habits hadn't changed, her waistline had expanded. Daily exercise was helping prevent serious poundage from accumulating. Still, she was roughly 10 pounds above her healthy weight and she was worried about gaining more.

At first, she tried to control her calorie and fat intake by measuring her foods, even her snacks. It helped, but still she wasn't satisfied with the results. She expected the pounds to come off much faster than they did. She decided that she needed to do something more.

Mary Ellen scrutinised her eating habits and quickly figured out that her problem wasn't what she was eating at home. "I travel a lot and I'm not a big fan of cooking, so I eat a lot of meals in restaurants," she explains. "You go out to these places and they just load you up with volumes of food. I was eating way too much."

So, she reasoned, why not be as diligent about portion sizes in restaurants as at home?

The next time she ate out, she gave the idea a try. When placing her order, Mary Ellen also asked the waiter for a doggie bag. And when both arrived, she didn't hesitate – she immediately divided the food into two portions, placing half in the bag.

Success! No longer tempted, Mary Ellen ate what was left on her plate and took the rest home.

This technique, along with a healthy diet and regular exercise, helped Mary Ellen take off those 10 pounds in about 6 months.

She has kept her weight in check ever since, no matter what's on the menu.

2 PLATES, 1 DINNER, MINUS 40 POUNDS

Jack Zimak and his wife believe in sharing everything, including dinner. This simple strategy helped him take off 40 pounds.

In 1997, at the age of 33, Jack went for his first physical in a long time. The news wasn't good. After years of not paying much attention to what or how much he ate, his weight had crept up to 17st 7lb. Worse, his cholesterol level had risen to well above normal. Jack thought of his father, who had died of a heart attack aged 60. He didn't want to risk the same fate.

"Like everyone, I needed motivation to change my lifestyle," says Jack, a sales manager. "My motivations were my cholesterol, my family history and my three kids. I wanted to be around to see them grow up."

Jack's doctor wanted him to get his cholesterol level down within 2 months and Jack rallied to the task. He gave up red meat, eggs, dairy products and fast food. He learned new ways to prepare fish and chicken, instead of frying them. His diligence paid off: when he had his cholesterol level rechecked 8 weeks later, it had dropped significantly. As a bonus, he had lost 15 pounds.

That initial weight loss inspired Jack to make more dietary changes. Mayonnaise was out, mustard was in. Butter was out, replaced by a bit of olive oil. Fizzy drinks and fruit juices were out, water was in.

Restaurants presented a bigger challenge. Jack and his wife, Jen, enjoyed eating out. But Jack knew that the gargantuan portions were no good for his physique. So the two of them got into the habit of ordering one main course and an extra plate. Then they'd split the food between the two of them. "Most restaurants were quite accommodating, especially when I showed them my driver's licence picture so they could see how much weight I had lost," Jack says.

How much did he lose? A total of 40 pounds in about a year. "My wife took off a few pounds as well," he reports.

Jack is content at his current weight of 14st 9lb, which he has maintained since 1998. To ensure that those extra pounds don't come back, he and his wife have started a daily walking programme. "And we still share our meals when we eat out," he adds.

WINNING ACTION ➤ ➤ ➤

Order one meal for two. *Restaurant meals are the downfall of many weight-conscious people. The portion-control technique that Jack uses is a great one for a couple of reasons. First, it immediately cuts your calories in half. And second, by eating with a fellow dieter, you have a built-in weight-loss buddy system.*

SHE NEVER LEAVES HOME WITHOUT HER LOW-FAT SPREAD

How can you lose 100 pounds on a 1,200-calorie-a-day diet and still enjoy going out to restaurants?

Carry individual portions of low-fat spread and fat-free salad dressing in your handbag. That's what Alayne Gunto did when she became determined to whittle down her 17st 4lb- figure.

Alayne comes from a family with a history of weight problems. While she tried on and off to slim down, she was never really successful. Then her mother, father and grandmother all had heart surgery within months of each other. That was the wake-up call Alayne needed. She decided to lose weight because, as she says, "I didn't want to put my husband and children through that experience."

Alayne put herself on a strict 1,200-calorie-a-day eating plan. She paid attention to what and how much she ate, something she had never done before. She kept close tabs on her portion sizes by reading food labels and using measuring cups. She started eating breakfast every day but quit her habit of munching on high-fat snacks. To bolster her resolve, she joined a slimming club where she participated in regular weigh-ins.

All of these strategies helped Alayne hold course on her self-styled weight-loss programme. But there is one trick in particular that has kept her from blowing her calorie and fat budget. "I like to eat out, but I want to know exactly what's going into my mouth," she explains. "I don't want to leave it up to the restaurant to tell me I'm eating low-fat. I don't necessarily believe their advertising. So I order my salads and baked potatoes plain. I just open my handbag and dress them myself."

Alayne's strategy worked. Within 15 months of starting her weight-loss programme, which included daily walks, she reached her goal weight of 10st 5lb. She has maintained this weight for 2 years.

These days, just looking in the mirror is incentive enough for Alayne, a 34-year-old homemaker, to keep her eating and exercise habits on track. And although she admits to occasionally going over her fat and calorie budget, she never goes to a restaurant without her condiments.

SHE WENT CASHLESS
AND LOST 50 POUNDS

Kathy Brown is 50 pounds lighter because she stopped carrying cash.

In 1994, at the age of 40, Kathy weighed 13st 3lb. And she knew why: she just couldn't resist those fast-food restaurants in her hometown. In fact, there were few days when Kathy *didn't* hit one fast-food joint or another. The greasy breakfasts were her favourites, though she ate more than her share of cheeseburgers and chips, too.

Disillusioned by gaining so much weight, Kathy decided that her fast-food feasts had to end. But giving up what had become an almost daily event wouldn't be easy. "I knew my weakness, so I had to figure out a way to overcome it," she says. Her solution was to leave all of her cash at home. She had her bank cards and credit cards to cover other expenses, but no money for food.

With fast foods all but gone from her diet, Kathy had to find something to fill the void. Vegetables and bread became her new dietary staples, supplemented by smaller amounts of fruits, dairy products and other proteins. "I never used to eat vegetables, never. I didn't even eat lettuce," she says. "Now, I eat all kinds of vegetables. My problem was that I had never tried them, so I assumed that I didn't like them."

These days, a typical meal for Kathy is stir-fried vegetables sprinkled with soy sauce and served over rice, with a baguette on the side. When she craves the convenience of fast food, she reaches for a low-fat frozen ready meal, instead.

By improving her eating habits, Kathy was able to trim 50 pounds from her 5-foot-5-inch frame. She's so confident of her ability to maintain her healthy weight of 9st 9lb that she has even relaxed her fast-food ban. She treats herself to whatever she wants, but only once every 2 weeks – on payday.

WINNING ACTION ➤ ➤ ➤

Detour around the fast-food route. Kathy found a unique way to break herself of the fast-food habit. In addition to travelling without cash (you may want to have some on hand in case of an emergency), you have a couple of other options. When you drive to and from work, use a route that doesn't pass by the local fast-food restaurants. And stock your glove compartment with non-perishable low-fat foods – pretzels, dried fruit, small boxes of cereal – to tide you over in case you get hungry.

SAVE NOW, SPLURGE LATER

Mary Adams longed for a way to enjoy the goodies at parties and holiday dinners without exceeding her 1,200-calorie-a-day limit. "I read that the average Christmas dinner has more calories than I eat in an entire day," says the 48 year old, who was restricting calories to slim down her 20st 6lb- frame.

Friends suggested that she try snacking on something before special eating events, but Mary doubted that would work for her. She feared that she'd eat beforehand and then indulge anyway, doubling her potential for gaining, rather than losing, weight. So she came up with the idea of banking calories.

"I realised that if I ate only 300 calories during the day, I'd have 900 left for dinner. I could eat what I wanted and not go over my calorie goal," she explains. "The trick was to find foods that would fill me up on the fewest calories." So she started checking her calorie counter for filling but low-cal foods. Among her choices were light bread, certain cereals, tiny crackers, carrots, celery sprinkled with chilli powder, sugar-free jelly and lots of water.

Like someone squirrelling away money from every pay cheque to buy an expensive coat or a new stereo system, Mary saves up calories so she can splurge on food at special events. "When my office planned a big holiday dinner, I saved 100 calories a day for 10 days," she says. "I was able to go to the dinner, sample all the great foods and not worry about overindulging!"

Since establishing her personal calorie account in 1998, Mary has dropped 8 stone. And she plans on using calorie banking to get to her 9st 9lb- goal. She's banking on making it.

WINNING ACTION ➤➤➤

Save, save, save, then splurge. While this tactic may not work for everyone, Mary found her own way to enjoy party foods without ruining her weight-loss efforts. As I say in my Ten Commandments of Weight Loss, slimming down doesn't have to mean giving up on all of the fun. You just have to find a way to do both. Give Mary's method a try to see if it works for you.

SHE NEVER GOES OUT ON AN EMPTY STOMACH

Shereen Tate discovered that eating a salad before she hit the party circuit put the brakes on her Christmas overeating – and her inevitable 5- to 10-pound weight gain at this time of year.

Normally, the 32 year old maintained good eating and exercise habits. She limited junk food, made sure she ate lots of fruits and vegetables and worked out regularly. Even when her last pregnancy left her with 20 pounds of "baby fat", she was able to take off the weight within a year, thanks to her healthy lifestyle.

Still, Shereen couldn't seem to get through Christmas without picking up a few unwanted pounds. Every year was the same: in the presence of savoury nibbles, tempting desserts and sparkling champagne, she would feel her willpower wane. By the time New Year arrived, Shereen found herself carrying some of the weight she had worked so hard to lose.

Shereen was able to take off the extra pounds, but she hated having to do it year after year. As yet another holiday season approached, she knew she had to find a way to stop herself from overindulging. Then it hit her: since she was most likely to eat too much when her stomach was empty, she'd make sure that her stomach was full *before* she started celebrating.

Shereen got into the habit of eating a pre-party plate of crisp lettuce topped with carrots, cucumbers and a splash of balsamic vinegar. She would leave her home with her tummy politely full. Once at the party, instead of lingering by the buffet table, she'd mingle with other guests. She'd sample a treat or two, but she didn't feel the urge to overindulge, as she had before.

Shereen's strategy worked like a charm. She survived that party season and seasons afterwards without gaining a pound. Now that's a cause for celebration!

WINNING ACTION ➤ ➤ ➤

Start social celebrations with a private mini-meal. Before heading to a party, help yourself to a snack to take the edge off your hunger. I like to grab a fruit bar before party time. It's easy and it's quick. Other good choices include a piece of fruit, yogurt or even a small plate of pasta.

HER PARTY STYLE KEEPS
HER AWAY FROM THE BUFFET

Socialising at parties kept Andrea Kennedy away from the buffet table and a lean 9st 9lb for more than 14 years.

Thin for most of her life, 51-year-old Andrea started gaining weight in 1980 after rupturing a disc while moving into a new home. The injury caused so much pain that she could hardly move. After undergoing surgery, Andrea was instructed to avoid exercise to prevent further injury. Her weight climbed from 9st 9lb to 10st 10lb, where it remained until September 9, 1985. That's when she joined Weight Watchers.

"Within 2 months, I was down to 9st 1lb," Andrea recalls. "But Christmas was around the corner and I could see that it had the potential to sabotage my hard work. I decided I needed a plan."

It started at her husband's company Christmas party. "As soon as I walked in, I did what I would usually do – head for the buffet table," she says. "Then I thought about how pleased I was with my weight loss." That stopped her in her tracks.

"I remembered that food wasn't the reason that I went to that party," Andrea says. "Friends were."

She scanned the room, found friends located away from the buffet table and struck up a conversation. When they migrated to the food Andrea found a new group to chat with. She avoided the buffet the entire night, a strategy she used to get her through the Christmas season. And it worked; she didn't gain an ounce.

Andrea eventually did gain back some weight. She felt too thin at 9st 1lb and allowed herself to go up to 9st 9lb. But she still follows her party ritual. "I spend my party time socialising," she says. "If I feel hungry, I scan the buffet table and decide what I want – low-fat only, of course. Then I send my husband to get it for me."

SHE LOST WEIGHT WITH BEN AND JERRY

Ten years ago, Karen Nitkin had a bedtime routine that was making her fat. Instead of sleeping, she would head to the kitchen and scoff down pints of Ben & Jerry's ice cream, frozen Snickers bars and spoonfuls of peanut butter. Today, the 32 year old is 40 pounds thinner, sleeps like a baby – and still eats Ben & Jerry's.

Her secret: she stopped starving herself.

After gaining 40 pounds during her first year of college, Karen was desperate to fit back into her smaller-size clothes. So she started dieting.

For breakfast, she'd eat a small bowl of cereal with skimmed milk. Lunch would be a small salad with just a dollop of dressing on the side. For dinner, she'd have a plain baked potato.

She'd struggle through the day, feeling hungry nearly all of the time. Late at night, hunger pangs would get the best of her and she'd raid the fridge.

The next day, she'd vow to do better. Breakfast would be a grapefruit; lunch, a pot of yogurt. Still not eating enough food during the day, Karen continued to binge at night. And the more obsessed she became with losing weight, the more she gained.

After graduating from college, Karen got a job as a newspaper reporter and met the man who would become her husband.

Together, they took long walks, played tennis and went for hikes in the woods. "Once I realised that he loved me despite my weight, I was able to start loving myself," Karen says. "I stopped obsessing about every bit of food that went into my mouth."

She began eating sensible meals – a bagel for breakfast, a sandwich for lunch, maybe some pasta for dinner. Fruit and yogurt became snacks, not meals. By eating healthy foods in sensible portions, Karen felt satisfied rather than hungry. Her night-time binges soon ended and the weight started coming off.

But Karen hasn't forsaken Ben & Jerry's. Only now, instead of eating a whole tub, she has a small amount and gives the rest to someone else.

WINNING ACTION ➤ ➤ ➤

Don't forbid yourself the foods that you love. Like Karen, one of the most important lessons that I needed to learn was how to enjoy "forbidden" foods without bingeing. Telling yourself that you can't eat certain foods is a sure way to set yourself up for a binge. If you follow the principles of my Ten Commandments of Weight Loss, you'll learn how to eat in moderation. That may sound foreign now, but you can change.

SHE'S NOW A THIN CHOCOHOLIC

Vicki Rogers Givens adores chocolate. She craves chocolate. She eats chocolate. And she has still taken off 5 stone.

How has she done it? By being choosy about her chocolate treats.

Ever since she was a child, Vicki, an administrative assistant, has fought the battle of the bulge. In college, she reached 16st 1lb, the most she has ever weighed.

These days, at 42, Vicki is a fit 11st 1lb. She says that she reached her goal weight by making smart food substitutions that save calories and still satisfy. For example, if she gets the urge to eat something salty, she chooses pretzels over crisps. In restaurants, she orders baked potatoes instead of chips.

Some of Vicki's smartest substitutions happen when those chocolate cravings hit. "Instead of high-fat chocolate chip biscuits, I eat a handful of chocolate rich tea biscuits," she says. That does the trick with far less calories and fat. Other favourites include fat-free chocolate pudding and hot chocolate.

It took Vicki only a year to hit her goal weight. She feels that she succeeded because she feeds her cravings instead of starving them. But she feeds them with smart choices.

Who says you can't outsmart a sweet tooth?

WINNING ACTION ➤ ➤ ➤

Want chocolate? Then eat! If you crave chocolate, go ahead and indulge. After all, this sweet treat may actually be good for you. According to researchers at the University of California, Davis, chocolate contains flavonoids, compounds that may help protect against heart disease. But try to stick with something low-fat and low-calorie, as Vicki does. You may yearn for a huge bowl of triple-chocolate-chunk ice cream, but low-fat chocolate yogurt with a drizzle of chocolate syrup will probably do the trick.

COLA JUNKIE GOES COLD TURKEY AND DROPS 30 POUNDS

When Maria Padron moved from the countryside to a big city in 1993, eating became a whole new experience. So was the weight gain that eventually followed.

"Food was everywhere," Maria recalls. "Fast food at every corner. Snacks anytime you wanted them. It was great."

What Maria got hooked on was not burgers, however. It was soft drinks. She drank 10 cans of sugar-laden cola a day. She went from a trim 9st 4lb to 11st 8lb in a year.

Then, she discovered that her cola habit was costing her 150 calories a can. At 10 cans a day, that was 1,500 calories a day or 10,500 calories a week!

Maria quit the colas cold turkey, trading them for calorie-free water. She also cut back on fried foods and started eating more fresh foods, especially fruits and vegetables, just like she used to do. And she took a full-time job as a nanny for triplets, which gave her plenty of exercise.

In 2 years, she was back to her former weight.

"I still drink at least eight glasses of water every day," says Maria, now 28. "Fizzy drinks don't cross my lips."

WINNING ACTION ➤ ➤ ➤

Can the cola. *One of the easiest ways to reduce your calorie intake is to substitute water or flavoured water for fizzy drinks and sugary fruit juices. What about diet drinks? Researchers at the Centre for Human Nutrition in Sheffield found that people who drink beverages loaded with artificial sweeteners such as aspartame actually eat more food.*

SOME FOOD FOR THOUGHT

You've probably heard that old admonition to think before you speak. Well, Sue McGovern thinks before she *eats* – and it has helped her maintain a 30-pound weight loss for 20 years.

Forty-two-year-old Sue never paid much attention to her food choices while she was growing up. "It was nothing for me and two or three of my friends to devour a huge tub of chocolate-almond ice cream and a 12-pack of doughnuts in a sitting," she says. "We didn't think of these episodes as binges. They were simply a way of life."

For Sue, that way of life eventually started showing on the scales. By the time she was ready to enter college, she weighed 12st 7lb. "But because I was tall and in reasonably good shape, I never looked fat – just big," she recalls.

In college, Sue didn't have a car, so she travelled everywhere via foot, bike or skateboard. To her pleasant surprise, she began losing weight without changing her eating habits. She was down to 11st 1lb when she graduated.

But once Sue started working full-time, her active lifestyle ground to a halt. "That's when I realised that I had to make better food choices if I didn't want to regain the weight that I had lost," she says. "I read all that I could about good nutrition and healthy eating and I changed my eating habits accordingly."

For the first time in her life, Sue began thinking about what she was putting in her mouth. She stopped eating for the sake of eating and instead chose foods with the greatest nutritional value. Red meat, crisps, chocolate and other high-fat, high-calorie foods disappeared from her diet. Grains, vegetables and tofu became her staples of choice. "I discovered all kinds of healthy foods that I'd never had before," she said. "I was intrigued by tofu, beansprouts and herbs. And I spent hours picking berries and wild nuts."

Through a combination of healthier eating habits and daily exercise – jogging was her activity of choice – Sue managed to take off another 10 pounds. Her weight has remained in the range of 10 stone to 10st 5lb for about 20 years.

HE SHED THE LAST 5, AT LAST

It took him 10 years to figure out how, but George Trott found a way to get rid of those stubborn last 5 pounds.

George, a computer consultant, was just about to turn 50 when he found out that he had diabetes and heart disease. "I wasn't really surprised, since both conditions ran on both sides of my family and I had been overweight for years," he says. But it was enough to motivate him to trim 40 pounds off his 6-foot-2-inch frame by eating more healthily and exercising regularly. "I didn't want a life of excess medications and insulin shots," he explains.

For years, he was happy about his new 13st 3lb-pound physique, but he knew he could lose a little more. At 58, he was still stuck with what he calls "4 or 5 pounds too much George."

On the suggestion of one of his grown-up kids, he visited Ann M. Chicchi, a registered dietitian. She looked at George's overall diet and exercise plan – which was good – and did some fine-tuning. She gave him a lower-calorie, low-fat eating plan that incorporated all of the nutrients that George needed. The plan also kept his carbohydrate intake at a level that was more appropriate for someone with diabetes and high triglycerides.

George took the food plan and moulded it to fit his eating

style. Instead of three large meals a day, he created a fourth small meal of whole-grain foods. "The complex-carbohydrate portion that Ann allotted for my breakfast I found more satisfying as a snack of whole-wheat crackers or bread around 9 o'clock at night," he says. He still had a good-size breakfast each morning, but he also had something low-fat and nutritious to nosh on before bedtime.

The result was that he finally shed those last few nagging pounds and his next blood count came back much improved as well.

So now, "4 or 5 pounds too much George" can call himself "just-right George".

WINNING ACTION ➤ ➤ ➤

When you hit the wall, call in a pro. If you're having trouble taking off those last few pounds, consider enlisting the help of a registered dietitian. To find one near you, contact your doctor or your local hospital for a referral. If group support is more your style, look in the Yellow Pages under "Dieting and Weight Control" for organisations such as Weight Watchers.

SHE GIVES HERSELF A DIET DAY OFF

Sandra Hameroff was having a hard time losing 40 post-pregnancy pounds – until she started taking time off from her diet.

Shortly after the birth of her son, Noah, Sandra got serious about shaping up, determined to return to her pre-pregnancy weight of 7st 2lb. She started using her cross-training machine four times a week. She also went on a strict diet, allowing herself no more than 1,300 calories a day and denying herself a lot of her favourite foods, especially pizza and chips. As a result, she found herself on the brink of a full-scale binge more than once.

When a sympathetic friend learned of Sandra's efforts – and her list of forbidden foods – she made a suggestion: "Why not give yourself a break from your eating programme once a week? You'll tame those cravings before they permanently undo your diet."

The next Monday through to Thursday, Sandra was a model of gastronomic self-control, amazing even herself. Then came Friday and with it, her old favourites: pizza, ice cream and a hearty dessert.

As radical as it sounds, indulgence was just what she needed. The next day, Sandra resumed her stricter eating plan with greater enthusiasm. Soon after, her husband got in on the act by taking her to dinner on Friday nights, which only served to make her splurges seem even more special. "I looked forward to them," she says. "They made my diet easier to stick with."

Four months later, Sandra stepped on the scales and discovered that she had lost all 40 pounds without guilt or giving up the foods that she loved. As a gift to herself, she hired a personal trainer to help her get in the best shape ever. "She brought me to a new level of fitness," Sandra says.

WINNING ACTION ➤ ➤ ➤

Give yourself a break. As we all know, dieting is hard work and temptation is everywhere. Instead of trying to fight the urge to splurge all the time, allow yourself a chance to indulge those fat fantasies every now and then. Just remember that you have to be on the wagon 6 days out of 7.

END EMOTION-DRIVEN EATING

SHE SHED STRESS –
AND 10 STONE – WITH TEA

Jeanette Green weighed more than 21st 6lb until she discovered the slimming power of tea.

After years of failed attempts to lose weight, Jeanette finally took control of her eating habits. She reduced her portion sizes and cut out junk food. Sure enough, the pounds started disappearing.

Although she was encouraged, Jeanette realised she still had one hurdle to overcome. While she ate healthily during the day, as soon as she arrived home from work, she'd be hit with the overwhelming urge to binge.

Like most of us, Jeanette felt tired at the end of the day. Just thinking of the chores and errands that she still had to do made her anxious and tense. To soothe herself, she would head straight for the refrigerator and grab the first food she saw.

Jeanette started thinking about her postwork behaviour and about a theme of the Overeaters Anonymous meetings that she had attended. The two seemed to tie together.

"Overeaters Anonymous doesn't concentrate too much on the food thing," Jeanette says. "The emphasis is on the head. They say that if you get your head straight, your body will follow."

Jeanette knew that her postwork binges were driven not by hunger but by her emotions. So she decided that instead of calming her nerves with food, she'd sip herbal tea.

As soon as she walked in the door in the evening, Jeanette would head straight for the kitchen and brew a cup of tea. Then she'd curl up somewhere quiet to relax and recharge for the evening. Her daily tea time became a treasured ritual as well as a means of stopping the munchies that threatened her weight-loss goals.

Jeanette, who's now 60, eventually lost 10 stone. And she has kept the weight off for more than 18 years.

> ### WINNING ACTION ➤➤➤
>
> **Sip tea to de-stress.** There's no question that stress is a big cause of weight gain. Find your own way to unwind, like Jeanette did. You'll probably find that a lot of things in your life – not just your waistline – will begin to come into better focus.

SHE QUIT HER BIG-TIME JOB AND LOST 85 POUNDS OF PRESSURE

For most of her life, Cindy Arvayo was an active person. Then, she started climbing the corporate ladder at a large electronics firm. "With that came all the stress," says Cindy, age 45. "I got into the habit of numbing out with food."

After about 13 years, her weight had crept up to more than 16st 11lb. She was working 70-hour weeks managing several manufacturing groups. Even though she never had time or energy to work out, she wanted and needed to be active. "I felt guilty that I wasn't, so I ate even more," she says.

Then one day, Cindy asked her husband a question that most men would never want to answer: "Does my weight bother you?" His thoughtful response turned Cindy's life around: "What I miss is being active and doing fun things with you."

"His words made me want to be a better woman," Cindy says. Her first step was to join a health club, where she took a beginner-level aerobics class. But she knew that wouldn't be enough to give her the healthy, balanced life she desired. So, 6 months later, she quit her job and went back to college to become a beautician. This wasn't a rash decision on Cindy's part. "I had accomplished everything that I had wanted to in my job and it was time for me to move on," she explains. "Having my own beauty business was a lifelong dream, so I decided to go for it."

With that single decision, Cindy unloaded much of the stress that had driven her weight gain in the first place. "It was the best thing that I ever did for myself," she says. She no longer felt the overwhelming urge to overeat. She got back to the active and athletic life that she had known before. Gradually, she lost 85 pounds.

These days, Cindy works just 3 days a week, operating her own skin-care centre. She's also training for her second sprint-triathlon, a race involving a roughly 1½-mile swim, a 20-mile bike ride and a 10k run. Most important, she's happy. "I made the choice to find the balance that was missing in my life," she says.

WINNING ACTION ➤ ➤ ➤

Find out what really matters. Like Cindy, so many of us are in jobs that we don't care about and we aren't doing the things that we love. We numb ourselves with food as a way of stuffing down our real emotions, desires and dreams. But life is short and we only live once. Draw courage from Cindy's victory and find out what's really important in your life. And as the saying goes, just do it.

SHE SHED 90 POUNDS OF EMOTION

In 1994, Melonie Heaton weighed 16st 1lb. She had no energy, could barely muster the stamina to climb the stairs at home and had no desire to socialise with her friends.

Today, Melonie weighs in at a svelte 9st 9lb. She slimmed down, she says, by learning to identify the emotional sources of her physical hunger.

Melonie, at 38, had been overweight for as long as she could remember. "I'd been on the weight-loss roller coaster, trying every diet on the planet to slim down," she says.

Then Melonie started walking for just a few minutes, a few days a week. "I was so physically out of shape that walking was the only thing that I thought I could tolerate," she explains. "I'll never forget my first walk. I was out of breath in 3 minutes. I had to be very patient with myself."

Her patience paid off. Those 3-minute, 3-days-a-week walks gradually got longer and faster and Melonie started dropping pounds. As a bonus, her energy level soared.

Inspired, she began looking for ways to improve her eating habits, too. Through what she calls a journey of self-exploration, she soon realised that she had fallen into a pattern of eating even when her body didn't really want food.

"I was misinterpreting feelings of fatigue, loneliness, dissatisfaction or low motivation as hunger," she recalls. "I discovered that in order to remodel myself outside, I first had to remodel myself inside."

Melonie learned how to face her feelings head-on and how to remedy them without food. Now, whenever she has the urge to eat, she asks herself what she *really* needs. Is her hunger genuinely physical? Or are her emotions calling out for sustenance? "If I realise that I'm bored, I get out a craft project or go shopping or find some other constructive way to occupy my time," she says.

By learning to distinguish between physical and emotional hunger, Melonie stopped eating for the wrong reasons. In 2 years, she lost 90 pounds. Now, even 3 years later, she can proudly say, "I no longer have a weight problem."

SHE FOUND HERSELF –
AND LOST 111 POUNDS

Coping with a fractured marriage and a satisfying but stressful job, Lynne Watson found joy in only one thing: eating.

Every morning, she'd head for the local bakery, where she'd pick up an apple turnover and two or three chocolate doughnuts. She'd polish them off before she got to work. For lunch, she'd eat pizza or a big sandwich, with biscuits for dessert. In the evening, she'd eat a Mexican dinner slathered with sour cream and guacamole.

While these foods made Lynne feel better, they also expanded her waistline. By 1985, she weighed 16st 6lb.

That year, Lynne spent Christmas Day alone. Despondent and desperate, she was at a crossroads. "The way I figured it, I could end my life or take control of it," she recalls. "I decided to grab control."

After much soul searching, Lynne ended her 19-year marriage and returned to college to complete her degree. "As I made these choices, I began to feel better about myself as a person," she says. "I began to feel empowered."

Her newfound self-assurance and self-esteem had another surprising benefit: she no longer experienced intense food cravings. "As I met new people, I relied on them, not food, for comfort and companionship," she says.

Through a combination of healthy eating and regular exercise, Lynne lost 111 pounds in 4 years. And she's happy to report that not one pound has come back. "I have no trouble keeping my weight under control," says Lynne, now 50 and a health-information manager and quality-improvement coordinator.

WINNING ACTION ➤➤➤

Nurture yourself without food. Feelings of loneliness, anger, sadness and frustration often trigger binges, says Marlene Schwartz, Ph.D., co-director of the Center for Eating and Weight Disorders at Yale University. If negative emotions prompt you to overeat, you need to find non-food ways to make yourself feel better. Try making a list of your favourite activities. Then, when you're in the mood for food, check your list to see what else you can do to make yourself feel even better. Try listening to your favourite music, pottering around your garden, reading a thriller or calling a good friend.

SHE UNLOADED HER EMOTIONAL BURDEN AND 268 POUNDS

When Sandra Youse was 23, her doctor told her that she would not live to see 50. At the time, she weighed 28st 8lb.

"Everyone in my immediate family is overweight," she says. "And in my extended family – among grandparents, aunts, uncles and cousins – there are lots of health problems. Heart disease, cancer and diabetes are pretty common."

Even with her doctor's dire warning, Sandra didn't get serious about slimming down until 10 years later. By then, she had gained almost another 100 pounds, reaching her top weight of 35st 1lb.

"In those 10 years, I had made some halfhearted attempts at dieting, but they weren't successful," Sandra recalls. "I reached a point where I was tired of being so heavy. And because of an inheritance, I finally had the money to do something about it."

In February 1997, she entered Structure House, a weight-loss facility about 90 minutes from her home. "I went there on the advice of friends who were familiar with the programme," she says. "They really believed that it could help me."

Sandra stayed there for 11 months. During this time, she received individual counselling to help her confront and cope with some painful issues from her past. "I learned that many people use food to avoid dealing with their problems and that I was one of those people," she says. "I had been overeating since I was a child."

As Sandra began to address her own issues and learn more positive ways of handling them, she was better able to control her eating habits. "Through counselling, I learned that eating couldn't solve my problems – that I had to find other ways of coping," she says. "I started talking with friends, telling them what I was thinking and feeling. If no one was available, I'd write down my thoughts instead.

"The ultimate goal of counselling is to resolve the underlying problem," Sandra continues. "That actually makes things harder for a while. There were times when I got so overwhelmed with my issues that I had to step back and take a break. But eventually, I'd move on."

By the time she left the residential programme in January 1998, Sandra had lost 138 pounds. She continued to follow the eating-

and-exercise guidelines that she had been given and once a week, she made the 90-minute drive to meet up with a counsellor. "Losing weight was tougher on my own," she says. "It definitely wasn't a straight line. I'd make some progress, then take a couple of steps backwards."

But Sandra was determined. In a little more than a year, she took off another 130 pounds, dropping to 15st 13lb.

Sandra, now 36, would like to lose another 70 or so pounds. To that end, she continues to eat healthily and exercise regularly and she sees a counsellor every week. The therapy is excellent, she says and it has helped her tremendously in dealing with the issues that contributed to her weight gain in the first place.

"People constantly tell me what an inspiration I am and how I give them hope," Sandra adds. "But I couldn't have done what I did if I hadn't learned to face my problems."

WINNING ACTION ➤ ➤ ➤

Take the big step, get help. Wow! Sandra's story is truly amazing – and inspiring. Whether it's a support group, an institute or a close friend, getting support and counselling in getting to the source of your problems is the first hurdle if overcoming overeating. If it worked for Sandra, it can work for you, too.

NOW 92 POUNDS LIGHTER, SHE'D RATHER READ THAN EAT

When thoughts of food draw Cynthia Herrmann towards the fridge, she distracts herself by grabbing a magazine or newspaper and heading for the sofa. This little trick has helped her ride out many a craving – and get rid of 92 unwanted pounds.

Cynthia didn't always have such control over her cravings.

They're one reason why her weight went over 14st 4lb – not once, but three times. The third time came as Cynthia neared her 40th birthday in 1991. "I had been losing and regaining ever since I was a teenager," she says. "Finally, I just got tired of having to wear size-24 dresses. I swore that I would lose the weight and keep it off."

At 16st 8lb, Cynthia figured that she had her work cut out for her. At first, she tried modifying her diet on her own. "I ate more fibre-rich foods, especially fruits and vegetables, because I knew they would fill me up faster," she says. "I chose lean meats and low-fat dairy products and I switched to healthier cooking methods."

The weight came off slowly but steadily and within 4 years, Cynthia plateaued at 12st 2lb. At that point, she decided to join Weight Watchers, where she learned to keep a food journal to monitor her eating habits. "Through the journal, I realised that I had a tendency to eat past the point of fullness," she says. Within 8 months, 30 pounds melted away.

Finally at her goal weight of 10 stone, Cynthia set aside her food journal – and the pounds started creeping back. "I wasn't eating well consistently and I started giving in to cravings again," she says. "I was better off when I wrote everything down."

But Cynthia didn't want to resume her journal. As much as it had helped her, it came to serve as a reminder of her missteps and mistakes. Discouraged, she searched for an alternative to rein in her cravings.

Cynthia believed that by distracting her attention at the first sign of a craving, she could buy time until she determined whether she was experiencing genuine physical hunger or emotion-based "head hunger". That's when she hit upon the idea of picking up a magazine or newspaper and forcing herself to read for 15 minutes. If she still felt hungry when she had finished reading, she would know that her body was demanding food and she'd eat. Often, though, she'd get so absorbed by what she was reading that 30 minutes would fly by – and when she had finished, her craving was gone.

Picking up a newspaper or the latest issue of a favourite magazine when she feels hungry has helped Cynthia, now 48, maintain her 10-stone figure for almost 4 years. "Taking the time to distinguish between physical and emotional hunger has made all the difference," she says. "I've learned to pay closer attention to *why* I want to eat and, when necessary, to address the real issue – be it stress or boredom or something else."

WINNING ACTION ➤ ➤ ➤

Pick up a juicy magazine instead of a juicy meal. When hunger is more mental than physical, divert your brain with a tempting book or magazine. Many times, I find that I'm just looking for a way to treat myself after a long day. I like to keep issues of fun magazines – Vogue or Vanity Fair – around to indulge myself. If you're still hungry after 15 minutes of reading, chances are, it's true hunger and you should eat.

HE LEARNED TO SAY NO TO FOOD

It took several painful years, but John DeGennaro, a 42-year-old van driver, discovered that a simple anti-drug slogan is as effective for weight loss as it is for substance abuse.

Addicted to cocaine, alcohol and nicotine, John joined Alcoholics Anonymous in 1994. Two years of hard work later, with support from both professionals and friends, he was clean.

When John stopped using, though, he noticed that food tasted better. How much better? Within a few short months, he gained 60 pounds. He was carrying 16st 8lb on his 5-foot-2-inch frame.

Unhappy, John sought help from a dietitian, who taught him how to make wiser food choices. It didn't help. John's problem was much bigger: he realised that he had become addicted to food. "Once I started eating, I couldn't stop," he says. "If I was offered a doughnut at a customer's office, I'd not only eat two more, but I'd hit every doughnut shop along my route."

Then he remembered: he had stayed clean from his drug addictions by avoiding places where drugs were available. He could do the same with food.

When John would drop off his packages, instead of sticking around, he would get back in his van. It was simple, but it worked.

John made other lifestyle changes that helped him control his food addiction and take off those unwanted pounds. Once again, he sought help from a dietitian – but this time, he successfully cut his fat intake and weaned himself off his favourite junk foods. He also launched an exercise programme that consisted of brisk walking as well as stretching and toning exercises. "It took a lot of discipline to stick with it, but I had a lot of support from my friends," he says.

Within 2 years, the extra pounds – 67 of them – melted away. Today, John maintains his weight at 11st 11lb. He wouldn't mind losing a few more, but he's not worried. He knows he can just say no to food.

WINNING ACTION ➤ ➤ ➤

Steer clear of food pushers. If colleagues offer you cakes or confectionery, graciously decline. Also, try to limit your time in break rooms and other common areas where cakes, biscuits and other temptations lurk. Sometimes, proximity beats the toughest willpower!

SHE'S DRESSED
FOR WEIGHT-LOSS SUCCESS

Julie Portner has a special fondness for chips, chocolate and biscuits. But she knows that eating too much of these foods isn't good for her figure. So when she's tempted to overindulge, she reminds herself about her wardrobe. In an instant, the temptation passes.

It was her wardrobe that first gave Julie the incentive to slim down. "Winter was coming on and none of my winter clothes fitted me any more," explains the 38 year old. "I wouldn't be able to wing it as I had done through the summer by wearing loose-fitting shirts and elastic-waisted shorts. But I wasn't about to go out and buy a whole new wardrobe, two sizes larger."

At 5 foot 2 inches and 19st 12lb, Julie wasn't obese, but she wasn't happy with how she looked or felt, either. "Some people asked if I was pregnant, because the weight came on so fast – about 17 pounds in 5 months," she says. "I was heavy and unfit and I felt unattractive."

Determined to begin losing the extra weight before winter arrived, Julie signed up for Weight Watchers in the autumn of 1996. The programme taught Julie how to make healthy food choices and control her portion sizes. It also persuaded her to exercise, inspiring her to walk for 40 minutes on an almost daily basis.

But what really made a difference, she says, was the programme's monthly weigh-ins. "They gave me incentive to continue eating healthily and exercising regularly," she explains.

Within 6 months, Julie lost 20 pounds. She looked trimmer and she felt better. But the real payoff came when her too-small winter clothes fitted comfortably again. "Actually, I reached my goal weight in April 1997, after winter was over," she says. "I made do that season by covering buttons and zippers that wouldn't close with baggy tops and sweaters. It was just good to know that my wardrobe would fit the next time that winter came around."

In the years since she shed the extra pounds, Julie has maintained her weight at 8st 6lb. She continues to eat healthily and exercise regularly, though occasionally she finds herself tempted by chips, chocolate or biscuits. In those situations, she reminds herself about how hard she worked to slim down and how nicely her wardrobe fits. Usually, that's enough to convince her to walk away.

"I've reached a point where my desire to continue fitting into my clothing is stronger than my desire to overeat," she says.

WINNING ACTION ➤➤➤

Let your clothes help you overcome a craving. You spy a tub of your favourite ice cream and you feel your willpower weakening. What to do? Try conjuring an image of your favourite dress or pair of jeans. Think about how nicely it fits and how good it makes you look or about how close you've come to being able to wear the garment after years of hanging it in the back of your wardrobe. Now, is that ice cream worth it? Probably not.

SHE PLAYS THE WAITING GAME

Verona Mucci-Hurlburt just loves the thick-cut chips that are served in the cafeteria of the building where she works. But the 38-year-old chiropractor knows that they're no good for her figure. So when she sees them on the menu, she employs a strategy that helps curb her craving. She tells herself that she can have them later.

Postponing her indulgences in this way helped Verona end her lifelong battle of the bulge and lose 60 unwanted pounds – permanently.

Certainly, she has come a long way since the days when she

carried 15st 2lb on her 5-foot-5½-inch frame. "I was chubby even as a small child," she recalls. "My mother put me on my first diet when I was just 4 years old." It was one of many that Verona would try over the years. "Usually, I'd lose some weight," she says. "But as soon as I went back to my old eating habits, the pounds returned."

Then, in 1994, Verona enrolled in Weight Watchers. "I knew other people who had been successful on the programme, so I decided to try it for myself," she explains. She attended weekly meetings, in which she learned all about food choices and portion control. "The programme gave me the structure and accountability that I needed to be successful," she says.

Newly enlightened on the subject of nutrition, Verona realised that her love of certain high-fat foods, especially pizza and chips, could jeopardise her weight-loss efforts. She tried hard to stay away from them, but as she recalls, "I let myself say yes way too often."

So she adjusted her game plan. Instead of forbidding herself her favourite foods, she simply delayed her indulgences. The thick-cut chips are a great example. "The cafeteria served them every 2 weeks," Verona says. "Instead of saying I couldn't have them, I'd tell myself, 'Wait until next time.' Two weeks later, I'd ask myself if I still wanted them. Sometimes, I did. Other times, I could pass them up."

The tactic worked so well that Verona applied it to other foods that didn't fit into her eating plan. "I had to know up front that I could eat the food sometime in the future," she explains. "The future could be 10 minutes away or 2 weeks away. The important thing was that I was taking time to think before I ate. That made all the difference."

With practice, Verona found that she could extend her waiting periods even longer. "I went from 10 minutes to tomorrow to a special event next month," she says. "I could pass up many fattening foods without feeling deprived."

And it shows. In just 9 months, Verona was 60 pounds lighter. She has maintained her weight at 10st 12lb ever since.

"For a woman of my stature, 10st 12lb may seem heavy," she observes. "But most of that weight is muscle because I've been doing strength training all along." In fact, she became so enthusiastic about exercise that she now teaches aerobics classes on the side. "Working out and learning to say 'later' to fattening foods keeps me trim and fit," she says.

WINNING ACTION ➤➤➤

Postpone your indulgences. Three cheers to Verona for coming up with a fabulous craving buster. By telling yourself that you can have a "forbidden" food at a later time, you can turn your back on temptation without feeling deprived. And when the appointed hour arrives, you may find that you can pass up the food that, a few minutes, hours or days ago, you couldn't live without. If you still want it, go ahead and indulge. At least you've thought about it first.

SHE SAVOURED THE FLAVOUR AND DROPPED TWO SIZES

Dina Jachens lost 40 pounds without giving up any of the foods that she craves. Instead, she learned to enjoy them one piece at a time.

Dina, a 31-year-old full-time mum, had her three children within 4 years. Each pregnancy left her a little bit heavier and she had an increasingly difficult time getting rid of the extra pounds. "I was busy every minute, but not doing the things I could have done to keep in shape," she says. "And I tended to eat whatever I could grab, which included lots of crisps and other salty snacks."

Even as her weight climbed towards 12st 7lb during those 4 years, Dina didn't think much about slimming down. Then, one day, as she sorted through some size 12 and 14 clothes that no longer fitted, she began thinking about a family reunion that she had recently attended. At past reunions, she had always received lots of compliments about her appearance. But not this time.

Dina looked in the mirror and took a good long look at herself. She didn't like what she saw. She vowed that she would get back into the size 10 that she had worn before having her kids.

"I realised that my eating habits had got out of control," Dina says. "I was eating whatever and as much as I wanted to. I'm a salt freak, so I'd eat crisps by the handful. And before my periods, I'd crave chocolate, so I'd eat a good part of a bag of M&M's."

Dina knew that she couldn't completely give up the foods that she loved. But she learned how to control how much of them she ate by savouring them one piece at a time. Take those M&M's. Dina stopped tossing them in her mouth a fistful at a time. Rather, she put one on her tongue and allowed it to completely melt before starting another. "It usually takes only about 10 M&M's until I feel satisfied," she says. "That's a lot better than a whole bag."

The same rule applied to crisps. Instead of eating them by the handful, Dina crunched one at a time, giving herself a chance to really savour the taste.

Dina made other changes in her eating habits, like giving up most desserts, and high-fat, high-calorie foods that she didn't really care for. "If there was something that I simply couldn't pass up, I'd eat only a bite or two, just to get the taste," she says. She also launched an exercise programme, walking 6 days a week.

In 12 months, Dina managed to take off 40 pounds. She's maintaining her weight at a healthy 9st 9lb – and she's back into her size 10 clothing.

SHE MAKES INDULGING FEEL LIKE A BIG EVENT

For Rosemary Chiaverini, weight loss and gain had been a lifetime struggle. "I tried everything short of getting my stomach stapled and my mouth wired shut," says 50-year-old Rosemary. In 1995, when she reached 17st 3lb, she decided to join Weight Watchers. There, she learned the principles of healthy eating and the tools for changing her eating habits. But she found that she needed some personalised strategies to make all that she learned work for her.

One of her strategies is to associate foods with special occasions. She eats hamburgers and hot dogs only at barbecues, popcorn only at the movies and pasta only on nights when she goes to the theatre. "I incorporate eating into the ambience of what I'm doing," she explains. "It gives the food officialness and meaning." It also gives Rosemary licence to indulge without going overboard.

On those occasions when she allows herself treats, Rosemary doesn't settle for inferior-quality foods. If she craves chocolate, she doesn't gobble down a cheap chocolate bar. She treks to a luxury shop, chooses six fancy chocolates and has them wrapped, two to a box. Then, she eats only one box at a sitting. Likewise, if she wants ice cream, she doesn't sit down with a tub and a spoon. She heads for the local café and has her favourite flavour served to her in a pretty dish. "All of this reminds me that I'm being good to myself, that I'm giving myself a gift," she says.

By turning her indulgences into events and using the portion-control skills and other tools that she learned through Weight Watchers, Rosemary lost 87 pounds in only 18 months. "This is the only thing that worked for me," she says. "I'm an emotional eater, so I had to change my mindset towards food. Now, when I think about food and losing weight, I don't think 'deprivation,' I think 'indulgence and pleasure.'"

WINNING ACTION ➤ ➤ ➤

Think quality, not quantity. Rosemary is really onto something here! Instead of taking a "sneaking" or "cheating" attitude towards indulging her cravings, Rosemary celebrates the pleasure of the occasional treat. Give yourself permission to do the same. Enjoy your favourite foods – buy the absolute best quality for yourself and savour every single bite.

SHE SWAPPED STRUDEL FOR CEREAL AND LOST 86 POUNDS

When Teresa Pucsek and her family moved from Hungary in 1951, Teresa took that country's tasty treats with her. She continued to make apple strudel, chicken paprika, goulash and dumplings. It kept her from feeling homesick.

It also made her overweight. In 1975, at 55, Teresa reached her top weight of 14st 9lb. "I was at a point where I just didn't like myself anymore," she says. "Then I read about Weight Watchers in a magazine and I decided to give it a try."

The programme taught Teresa how to make smart food choices and how to cook with low-calorie ingredients. "I was amazed at how quickly the pounds began to disappear," she says. "I lost between 7 and 8 pounds in the very first week."

But then, Teresa noticed that her weight loss was slowing down. She did an inventory of what she was eating and found one culprit showing up repeatedly – her favourite, apple strudel. She was indulging once or twice a week.

"You keep eating what you grew up with," Teresa says. "It's built into you. So I had to figure out a way to eat differently but still get that familiar, old-home feeling."

Teresa decided to trade her strudel for cereal. She had a bowl every evening, before she went to bed. The sugar in the cereal satisfied her sweet tooth as the strudel once had. And the milk, which she drank while growing up in Hungary, reconnected her with her childhood. She was able to lose weight without feeling deprived.

Teresa, who's now 80, shed a total of 86 pounds in about a year and has kept off the weight for 24 years. These days, she teaches baking at her local adult education centre, where she occasionally whips up a batch of her apple strudel. She even allows herself a serving, as a treat. But she hasn't forsaken her bedtime snack of cereal, creating her own concoction of one sugary brand and three nonsugary brands. "I constantly alter the proportions so that the mixture always tastes a little different," she explains.

WINNING ACTION ➤ ➤ ➤

Satisfy your sweet tooth with a new favourite. A bowl of cereal with skimmed milk can satisfy a craving for sweets without blowing a healthy diet. Like Teresa, I satisfy my nighttime cravings for sweets with cereal, but without milk.

HE TUNED OUT HIS BAD HABITS

After battling a weight problem for most of his life, Mark Maron tuned in to the surprising, binge-fighting power of music and successfully shed 25 pounds.

Mark first got serious about slimming down and staying healthy in 1997. That's when at the age of 34, he found out that his mother had breast cancer. "I realised that both my mother and I had to start eating smarter – me, to lose weight and avoid getting cancer; her, to possibly save her life," he explains.

Mark, who weighed 18st 13lb at the time, read as much as possible about health, nutrition and fitness and tried to incorporate all that he learned into his life. For him, that meant eating more vegetables and fruits, trying to steer clear of fatty foods and working out at the gym at least three times a week.

Sure enough, the extra pounds melted away. But that wasn't the end of Mark's weight problem. It seemed that when he had some kind of emotional upset – a crisis at work, a fight with a loved one or another problem that made him feel bad – he would binge on high-fat foods. "I would feed my emotions by eating things from fast-food restaurants and pizza houses, then go straight to bed when I got home," he recalls. Needless to say, overeating only made Mark feel worse and he found himself trapped in a vicious cycle.

During a down moment one day, Mark found himself heading for one of his fast-food haunts. Then he remembered a song that he had heard on the radio just a few hours before and decided to make a stop at the nearest music store. "I picked out two CDs. One was by a band called Big Audio Dynamite and the other was an assortment of 1970s tunes, including my favourite, 'Born to Be Alive,'" he recalls. "The music was very high energy and upbeat. It really pumped me up." He got so pumped up that he forgot about stuffing down his sorrows with food and headed for the gym instead.

It's a habit that has stuck with him ever since. Whenever he senses a slump coming on, Mark cranks up the tunes. Sometimes, he goes to the gym and works out; other times he just stays home and dances. "I danced a lot of my weight off," he says.

In fact, by autumn 1998, those 25 unwanted pounds that Mark had carried around for so long finally disappeared. He maintained his weight at 17st 2lb for several months before enrolling in a personal coaching programme. Now he's down to a muscular 16st 6lb and he hopes to lose a little more. "My mum is better now and we're both living healthier than we ever have," he says. "We're feeling great about it!"

WINNING ACTION ➤ ➤ ➤

Tune in to fun instead of food. Like Mark, we all hit speed bumps that can send our egos and self-esteem plummeting and trigger a binge. Keep a "fun list" around so that when you get knocked off your feet by something, you can turn to a positive source of consolation, rather than to a tub of ice cream.

---

87 POUNDS GONE THROUGH THE POWER OF PRAYER

Devoutly religious, Theresa Giffin says that her relationship with God has been her salvation from a lifetime of weight problems.

"I had tried everything available to lose weight," she notes. "I took pills. I fasted. I got a tummy tuck. I did it all. And each time, I'd regain what I lost – and more."

But for Theresa, prayer succeeded where pills, fasts and surgery had failed. It happened one day when a colleague left a box of chocolates on her desk.

Theresa took one piece, but she knew that wouldn't be

enough. "It was my very favourite and I thought I wouldn't be able to stop," recalls the 51-year-old nurse. "So I whispered a little prayer: 'God, you know that I want to eat this whole box of chocolates. You have to help me!'"

In an instant, Theresa's desire for chocolate vanished. "It had no smell, no taste," she says. "It was like a piece of cardboard to me."

Theresa joined Weigh Down Workshops, an international programme that advocates weight loss through prayer. She credits this approach with her weight-loss success.

Now, every time temptation hits, Theresa says a little prayer. In little more than a year, she lost 87 pounds.

WINNING ACTION ➤ ➤ ➤

Create your own intervention. When you feel that overwhelming surge of emotions sending you off on a binge, stop it in its tracks. Like Theresa, you can pray. Or you can do what I do: before I start stuffing myself with food, I say to myself (or sometimes out loud), "Stop, slow down and think!" Usually, that's enough to help me switch gears, so I can do something – anything – else.

THE PEN IS MIGHTIER THAN THE FORK

As the owner of an agency that provides makeup artists for stage actors and TV personalities, 37-year-old Juanita Dillard was constantly surrounded by thin, gorgeous women – and free buffets. The ever-present food proved to be too much of a temptation for Juanita, especially in such a high-pressure environment.

"I'd eat all day, then help the caterers clean up just so I could take home the leftovers," she says. Before she knew it, she weighed 19st 8lb.

It took a souvenir photo from a holiday in the Cayman Islands to persuade Juanita to slim down. "The photo was taken in late 1989. When I saw how I looked, I became determined to lose weight in the new year," she says. "I was tired of compliments that stopped at my face. There I was, surrounded by gorgeous women. I wanted to be one, too."

Juanita stopped heading for the big buffets and instead signed up for Weight Watchers, where she learned about portion control and the importance of filling up on vegetables. But the most valuable lesson she learned was how to keep a journal. When she started writing about her stress instead of feeding it, the weight rolled off. In a year-and-a-half, she lost 137 pounds.

The biggest test of her weight-loss success came when her dog, Nikki, was killed by a car. Distraught, Juanita grabbed a block of cheese, a jar of black-bean salsa, a super-size bag of tortilla chips and a bottle of wine – all the fixings for a binge. Before long, tears were rolling down her cheeks. The jar of salsa was empty; the bag of tortillas, half-eaten.

By chance, Juanita reached into her bag and felt her journal. She took it out and started writing about how much she missed Nikki. When she was through, she felt better and her desire to eat was gone.

"Stress was what made me fat before and I wasn't going to let it happen again," she says. "Now, keeping a journal is my zero-calorie stress buster."

WINNING ACTION ➤ ➤ ➤

Put your feelings on paper. The next time you're inclined to pick up a fork, grab a pen instead and start writing. Research shows that keeping a journal when you're tense can help avoid emotional eating.

MEDITATION:
AN AMAZING
FOOD SUBSTITUTE

Angela Banks turned to meditation to help her cope with stress and negative emotions. She never imagined that it would also help her lose 50 pounds.

For years, Angela used food to block out memories of her painful, unhappy childhood. Eating made her feel warm and fuzzy inside. It was her way of showing herself kindness and love. But it came at a price: by the time she reached her twenties, she weighed 13st 6lb.

All the while, Angela's emotional pain continued to fester inside her. It finally came to a head in an explosive confrontation with her husband.

At that moment, Angela realised that she could no longer ignore what had happened to her as a child. It was not only driving her to overeat, it was also undermining her spiritual well-being as a mother, wife and business owner.

Angela immediately sought professional help. She learned an array of coping skills, including meditation. Now, instead of running to the refrigerator when she feels bad, she heads for a quiet room.

For a few minutes, she tunes out the outside world and tunes in to her innermost thoughts and emotions. She tries to identify what is really bothering her, then figures out how to deal with the real problem without turning to food.

Today, at 34, Angela runs a non-profit organisation that provides personal counselling and career support for sexually abused women. She credits a combination of meditation and prayer with helping her turn her life around.

It also helped her slim down: she maintains a healthy weight of 9st 12lb.

HE'S NO LONGER THE BIG MAN ON CAMPUS

As college athletics trainer, Stephen R. Nemes Jr. has made a career out of getting student athletes into top shape for their respective sports. Sometimes, that means helping them lose a few pounds, an assignment with which Steve has had plenty of personal experience.

In 1975, Steve, then a college second-year, reached his top weight of 17st 9lb. "I had been heavy even as a child, but I really let myself go as a teenager," he says. "I ate a lot of junk food and I didn't exercise nearly enough."

At 5 foot 5 inches, he couldn't conceal his girth. Yet he remained unfazed by his portliness until one of his professors confronted him about it. "He told me that I might have a hard time finding a job as an athletics trainer because I was so overweight," Steve says. "Employers wouldn't view me as a credible candidate." The professor's comments left Steve shaken. His dream was to train athletes. He wasn't about to let his weight get in the way.

Of course, slimming down in a college environment, where junk food is plentiful and watching TV is a popular pastime, presented its own challenges. "My problem was that whenever I had some downtime, I'd sit in front of the TV stuffing myself with whatever I could get my hands on," Steve says. "I was overeating and under-exercising."

He made an effort to fill his free time with other activities, like working out, shopping for healthy foods and studying. "As my weight went down, my grades went up," Steve says. By the time he graduated in 1977, he was 82 pounds lighter.

In the years since, Steve's weight has fluctuated between 11st 11lb and 12st 7lb. He tries to stay fit to set a good example not only for the student athletes he trains but also for his family. "I have a little girl whom I want to see grow up," he says. "She has become my biggest motivator.

WINNING ACTION ➤ ➤ ➤

Fill up your downtime. All of us have moments when we just want to lie back and watch the world go by. That's fine . . . once in a while. There are plenty of ways to relax without even thinking about food. Get a facial. Play fetch with your dog. Take a class in garden design or bird-watching. Buy a telescope and watch the stars. You get the idea. Eating is often a response to boredom. If you aren't bored, you won't eat.

SHE BIKED AWAY
FROM BINGEING

Joanie Morris knows all too well what loneliness can do to her appetite and her waistline.

In September 1996, Joanie, then a regional manager for a health-care company, had to leave her family for a 1-year job assignment at company headquarters, hundreds of miles away from home. Every evening, while her colleagues were enjoying the company of family and friends, she'd sit by herself in the small flat that her employer had provided. She'd read and watch television until about 7:30 p.m., when she'd call her husband and daughter.

"Usually, after I hung up the phone, I'd just sit and cry," Joanie recalls. "I missed my family so much. I could see them only on weekends – and not every weekend, at that. It was incredibly lonely."

For comfort, she began treating herself to dinner at a little Italian restaurant. "My flat had a kitchen, but I thought that going out was easier," she explains. "I'd eat a snack when I got home from work, then go over to the restaurant after talking to my family." Needless to say, she got to know the menu very well. "I especially loved the large pasta dishes with creamy, cheesy sauces," she says. After dinner, she'd return to her flat, where she'd help herself to a bowl of ice cream and some biscuits.

While this ritual made Joanie feel better, it also took a toll on her figure. In just 3 to 4 months, she gained 20 pounds. "One weekend, a friend of mine said to me, 'You may not like your job, but you sure must like the food,'" she recalls. "I was mortified. When I stepped on the scales, they read 10st 2lb. I had never weighed that much – except when I was pregnant."

As she headed back to her job in January 1997, Joanie resolved to start a new after-work routine that would put an end to her nightly binges and help her slim down. As soon as she arrived at her flat, she'd change her clothing and head straight for her building's fitness room. There, she'd put in an hour on the treadmill and exercise bike while watching the evening news. Then, she'd return to her flat, shower and call her family.

"Even though I was exercising to lose weight, I noticed that I felt better, too," Joanie says. "The physical activity seemed to lift my sadness and even out my moods."

Joanie also cut back on her nightly forays to the Italian restaurant next door, instead stocking her kitchen with healthy staple ingredients for fast and easy dinners.

Between her improved eating habits and her nightly exercise routine, Joanie was able to get rid of the 20 pounds that she had gained, plus a few more. She returned home at the end of her job assignment weighing 8st 7lb, where she's stayed ever since.

"I was determined to slim down by the time my assignment was over and I did," says Joanie, now a 41-year-old full-time mum. "I think that exercising made the difference. It helped me emotionally as well as physically."

WINNING ACTION ➤ ➤ ➤

Boost your mood without food. Feeling blue? Instead of heading for the fridge, put on your trainers for a few minutes of physical activity. Research has shown that exercise can improve your mood by triggering the release of endorphins, opiate-like brain chemicals that can make you feel good all over. You'll avoid a binge and you'll burn some calories to boot.

GET YOUR
BODY MOVING

FROM THE CLOSET
TO THE WINNER'S CIRCLE

Do you remember what you were doing on November 4, 1980?

Sharon Turrentine does. It made her the slim, strong woman that she is today.

On that particular day, Sharon was lying in bed, watching TV and eating chocolate. At 36, she was unhappy and feeling sorry for herself. Her son was about to get his driver's licence and she felt that she wasn't needed anymore. Then there was her weight: at 5 foot 2 inches and 9st 6lb, she dressed in the closet to avoid looking at her body.

As Sharon nibbled on her chocolate and brooded about her life, the images on the TV screen grabbed her attention. It was the first-ever Ms. Olympia Bodybuilding Competition. As she watched the women show off their strong, shapely physiques, Sharon snapped out of her funk. "I announced to my husband, 'I'm going to be a bodybuilder,'" she recalls.

The very next day, Sharon – who had not exercised in years – dug out an old leotard and headed for the local gym. Gradually, she established a regular workout routine using information she had gathered from books and magazine articles on weight training.

"When I first started out, I couldn't climb a flight of stairs without being out of breath. Five pounds was the most I could lift," Sharon says. "Now, I bench-press more than 100 pounds."

To support her exercise programme, Sharon made some changes in her diet, too. "I remembered all the nutrition information that I had learned at school, such as the basic food groups and proper portions," she says.

Within 3 years of starting her exercise programme, she dropped four dress sizes. And Sharon, a woman who had once dressed in the closet, was ready to show off her 7st 11lb-pound body in competition. Over the next 7 years, she entered a number of bodybuilding contests. She collected a total of 15 trophies, never placing less than second. "I was old enough to be my competitors' mother," she adds.

Now, at 55, Sharon runs her own business, teaching other women how to lift weights and shape their bodies. "I want to set an example," she says. "I want them to know they can do this."

WINNING ACTION ➤ ➤ ➤

Show off your accomplishments. Sharon's quite an achiever! But don't feel you have to try out for the Ms. Olympia competition to get a sense of accomplishment. Training for any special event – a 5k run, a swimming competition, a bicycle race – will give you something to strive for. It will also motivate you to stick with a regular workout routine. If you're not into competition, do it for charity. Many non-profit organisations raise money through non-competitive athletic events.

PERSONAL MOTTO LED TO 125-POUND WEIGHT LOSS

When Tawni Gomes stopped making excuses, she started losing weight – almost half of her body weight, in fact.

Tawni's epiphany came one day in September 1996 as she watched *The Oprah Winfrey Show* on television. Oprah's guest was her personal trainer, Bob Greene. As Greene explained the basics of weight loss to the audience, Tawni began to feel inspired. At 21st 6lb, she knew that she had to slim down. So she headed for the nearest bookshop and picked up a copy of *Make the Connection*, Winfrey and Greene's book. She read it from cover to cover that very night.

Over the next month, Tawni struggled to stick with the exercise programme. Excuses like "There aren't enough hours in the day" and "I don't have a personal trainer" conveniently prevented her from making a serious commitment to slimming down.

Then she heard that Greene was coming to town to speak and do a book signing. Book in hand, she went to hear him. "A woman in the audience asked Bob how she was supposed to find time to exercise with four kids, a house and a full-time job," she said. "Bob looked her straight in the eye and without hesitation said, 'You're not ready to lose weight.' He turned to the rest of the audience and said, 'Next question.'"

Tawni's jaw dropped. "I was so shocked by his bluntness. But I had to admit that I was making the exact same excuses," she says. "Everybody has the same number of hours in a day. If people with kids and tighter schedules than mine can find time to exercise, then, I figured, so can I."

The very next morning, Tawni rolled out of bed at 4:00 a.m., laced up her walking shoes and headed out – alone – for a brisk walk. It was the start of what would become a daily ritual. "With my work schedule and family commitments, that was really the only time I had to exercise," she says. "At that early hour, it was so quiet and peaceful that it gave me a chance to think about my life and clarify my goals."

Over time, Tawni switched from brisk walking to running. She also began lifting weights and performing stretching and toning exercises. The combination enabled her to take off 125 pounds in 3 years.

"No excuses" remains Tawni's life motto. At 34, she continues to work out regularly and her weight is holding steady at 12st 7lb. "That's about right for my height and bone structure, though I'd like to lose about 20 more," she says. She now has an on-line support group to help others get on the road to "no excuses".

WINNING ACTION ➤ ➤ ➤

Make time, not excuses. We all have things that we need to get done, so we end up doing what's important to us. Decide what's most important for you. When you make yourself and your desire to live a healthier life a top priority, that's when weight loss will happen for you.

FROM MATRONLY
TO MARATHONER

Marlene Dropp was so out of shape that she couldn't even walk around the block. Seven years later, at 51, she walked a marathon.

A veteran dieter, Marlene had struggled with her weight all of her life. Sometimes she'd lose a few pounds, but they would always come back.

Then one day, as she looked in the mirror, Marlene realised how much she disliked the image that she saw. "I was a frumpy 14st 4lb- matron," says the mother of four. "My dress had stripes, a frilly collar and fluffy sleeves, like something my mother would have worn. I couldn't fit into more fashionable clothes. That's when I started feeling like a blimp."

That's also when she decided to do something about it.

Because of her weight, Marlene felt too self-conscious to exercise in public. But this time, she was determined.

So one beautiful morning in 1989, with her husband at home

to watch the kids, Marlene decided on impulse to take a walk around her neighbourhood. To her surprise, she arrived home energised. "That's when I decided to make walking part of my daily routine," she says.

Immediately, Marlene set a goal for herself. She wanted to advance from walking around the block to walking 5 miles a day. Her neighbourhood is laid out in half-mile circles, so she just kept adding circles to her route. Within 2 months, she achieved her goal. So she set her sights on a new objective: she wanted to cover a mile in 13 minutes. A year later, she could do it with ease.

Within 2 years of starting her exercise programme and making some changes in her eating habits – primarily avoiding fats and sweets – Marlene lost 50 pounds. As she got faster, she began entering walking races – 1-mile, 2-miles and 5k. In 1996, she celebrated her 51st birthday by entering a marathon. She completed the 26-mile course in less than 6 hours.

Even though she continues to compete, Marlene credits those daily walks around the block with jump-starting her weight-loss efforts. Today, at 55, she maintains a healthy weight of 10st 10lb.

WINNING ACTION ➤ ➤ ➤

Follow the 10 per cent rule. Just as Rome wasn't built in a day, neither is an exercise programme. Whatever activity you choose – walking, running, cycling, swimming or something else – start slow and easy. Gradually build to your desired duration and intensity. A good rule of thumb is to increase your level of activity by 10 per cent a week. So if you're able to walk for 10 minutes your first time out, stay at that level for 1 week. Then add 1 minute – 10 per cent – to your workout the next week. Continue until you're walking for 30 minutes a day.

SHE TOOK A DEEP BREATH AND LOST 215 POUNDS

LisaKay Wojcik was so overweight and out of shape that even 2 minutes' worth of exercise left her so breathless that she feared she'd have a heart attack. But finding the way to breathe correctly helped put her at ease to do the exercise that eventually helped her lose 215 pounds and regain her self-respect.

LisaKay, watched her weight climb to 23st 3lb through two tumultuous marriages. The combination of personal upheaval and unhealthy weight gain left her an emotional wreck. "I had no self-esteem left," she says.

But LisaKay believed in an old but true cliché. When things get that bad, there's only one way to go: back up.

"I wasn't emotionally prepared to tackle the problem with my marriage, but I believed that I could improve myself," LisaKay says. So she went out and bought a low-impact aerobics video and started work. "After just 2 minutes, I was sweaty, beetroot red and breathless," she says. "I thought I was going to die."

Convinced that she was having a heart attack, LisaKay called for an ambulance. "When I got to the hospital, the doctor tersely told me that I was merely out of breath," she recalls. "And to warm up next time." Too embarrassed to try aerobics again, LisaKay switched to a seemingly simpler activity: walking. Her first time out, she walked one-quarter mile so slowly that it took 40 minutes. Three months later, she could do 1 mile in an hour.

Six months later, LisaKay was ready for a more intense challenge: a "fat-burner" aerobics video. With her legs kicking high in the air and her arms moving nonstop, she was unaccustomed to such high oxygen demands – and that heart attack scare returned. Back to the hospital she went.

This time, a different doctor said she was breathing incorrectly. "He told me to breathe in through my nose and out through my mouth while exercising," she says. "He said to exhale harder to force a deeper inhale, since this sends more oxygen to muscles."

That simple tip did the trick. LisaKay continued exercising, gradually adding light weight training and toning and stretching exercises to her workout routine. She made some dietary changes as well, trading in fatty fried foods for salads, steamed cauliflower and water-packed tuna. Within 1 year, she had lost 75 pounds. Two years later, she had shed a total of 215 pounds.

Today, at 33, LisaKay is holding steady at 7st 12lb. She has joined a fitness club, where she works out on the treadmill and weight machines. At home, she does lots of marching on the spot, along with exercises to strengthen and tone her body.

Determined to use her life lessons to inspire other overweight women to improve their lives, LisaKay has become a motivational speaker and counsellor. "I learned that I matter," she says. "My message to others is that they matter, too."

WINNING ACTION ➤ ➤ ➤

Learn how to breathe before you keel over. Exercise increases your need for oxygen. To meet the demand, you need to breathe deeper. Here's how: stand with your feet shoulder-width apart. Keep your knees slightly bent, your pelvis tucked in and your chin parallel to the floor. Relax your shoulders and let your arms hang at your sides, with your elbows slightly bent and your fingers relaxed. Inhale slowly and deeply through your nose for a count of four and as you do, feel your abdomen extend. Then exhale slowly through your mouth for a count of four, feeling your abdomen return to its normal position. This will not only prevent you from becoming light-headed during exercise, it may lower your chance of getting stitches or cramps.

SHE RUNS TO READ –
AND LOST 68 POUNDS

Rebecca Harding wasn't always an exercise buff. In fact, 49-year-old Rebecca used to shy away from most physical activity because she was too ashamed of her size. Now, she's an avid runner, sometimes going out twice a day. And she's 68 pounds lighter.

What transformed this former couch potato into a fitness fanatic? She credits audio books.

"I was always much heavier than I wanted to be," Rebecca says. "As a teenager, I was 30 pounds overweight." Through marriage and three pregnancies, she continued to gain. By 35, she weighed 14st 8lb.

All the while, Rebecca's self-esteem plummeted. She began avoiding social events and even dreaded food shopping, for fear that she'd run into someone she knew who'd notice how much she had gained. "All I wanted to do was stay home and eat," she says. "The more I ate, the worse I felt about myself. The worse I felt about myself, the more I ate."

Rebecca's turning point came the day she waited in a hospital casualty department with one of her sick children. "A nurse asked me when my baby was due," she said. "I was mortified. I wasn't pregnant." she says. "Then and there, I made up my mind to slim down."

Out went the junk food and fast food, replaced by healthy choices such as whole-grain cereals for breakfast, salads for lunch and skinless chicken breast – stir-fried in lemon juice instead of oil – for dinner.

For exercise, Rebecca joined a local walking group. As she got trimmer and fitter, she went out on her own, graduating to jogging and eventually to running.

Rebecca enjoyed the faster pace of her workouts, but she missed the companionship of her walking-group friends. To keep herself from getting bored, she decided to listen to audio books while she ran. "I had used the tapes occasionally while I was driving and I enjoyed them immensely," she explains.

She began borrowing tapes from her local library and listening to them during her workouts. "I told myself that I could play them only when I was running," she says. "If I got really caught up in a particular tape, I'd run twice in one day just to finish it."

That may explain why she was able to lose 68 pounds in just 8 months. Fifteen years later, she maintains her weight at 9st 10lb. And she continues to eat healthily and run daily, always with her audio books in tow.

"Just recently, I ran to a tape of *The Horse Whisperer*," Rebecca says. "Later, when I drove my route to measure it, I couldn't believe how far I had gone. Almost 9 miles up a steep hill – and in the rain. I hadn't even noticed because I was so into the tape."

WINNING ACTION ➤➤➤

Catch up on your reading while you work out. Listen to audio books, available at most libraries, while you run, walk or do other types of exercise. The stories will keep your mind occupied and you'll finish your workout before you know it. In fact, you may even find yourself looking forward to your next session. A word of caution, however: if you live in an area where there's lots of traffic, you may want to leave your headphones at home. You need to know what's going on around you, for safety's sake.

THIS EARLY BIRD CAUGHT THE POUNDS-OFF PRIZE

At 42, LaVonnia "Bonnie" Johnson weighed 16st 1lb and wore a size 24 dress.

Then she started getting up earlier in the morning – and she lost 65 pounds.

Heavy all her life, Bonnie, put on even more weight after going through a painful divorce. But her life changed in 1993 when she read an inspiring story of a woman who had left a troubled marriage and thrived. That was just what Bonnie needed to hear. "If she could do it, I can, too," Bonnie thought.

In the beginning, she tried simple workouts – swimming, cycling and treadmill walking – at different times of the day, fitting it in whenever possible. And she made some progress, losing 15 pounds within 18 months.

Then Bonnie changed jobs. Her new work schedule was so erratic that she could exercise only in the early morning. For Bonnie, that turned out to be the turning point.

At 6:00 a.m., Bonnie would arrive at her local gym and head straight for the treadmill, stairclimber or exercise bike. Before long, she was experimenting with strength training. She was hooked. She couldn't begin her day without hitting the gym. Within 2 years, she lost 65 pounds and four dress sizes.

Today, at 49, Bonnie still starts her day with exercise. "Morning exercise has become a way of life for me," she says. "It's like drinking water or breathing. I need it to survive."

WINNING ACTION ➤ ➤ ➤

When it comes to exercise, be an early bird. Like Bonnie, make exercise the first item on your daily agenda. Starting my day on the treadmill is the only way that I know I'll fit in my workout. You'll rev up your metabolism so you burn more calories over the course of the day. As a bonus, you'll feel more centred, energised and better able to handle stressful situations.

EXERCISE TOPS HER TO-DO LIST

As an attorney, Sarah Yerger's day is jam-packed with meetings and other appointments. But she always saves her final appointment for herself: she heads for the gym. Scheduling her workout time in this way has enabled her to melt 55 pounds off her 5-foot-4-inch frame.

Like everyone else in her family, Sarah had always been overweight. "I believed that I was destined to be that way, so I didn't pay attention to my food choices or exercise as much as I should," explains the 31 year old. And it showed: over the years, her weight crept towards 14st 4lb.

Then Sarah's mother developed health problems because of her excess weight. Shaken by her mother's poor health, Sarah felt that her own weight might put her at risk of illness in later years. So she decided to do something about it.

Her first step was to join a local gym. But with her hectic work schedule, she had a hard time keeping her promise to go every day. That's when she came up with the idea of adding her workouts to her appointment calendar.

Keeping those exercise appointments isn't always easy. "But even on the busiest days, I make every effort to get to the gym," Sarah says.

Sometimes, special occasions – like a party for a friend's birthday or a colleague's promotion – coincide with Sarah's scheduled workout time. On those days, she simply plans her workouts for the morning. She arrives at the celebrations feeling good that she didn't shortchange her health.

But when she receives a spur-of-the-moment invitation to join her colleagues for an after-work happy hour, Sarah politely declines. "I always say no without feeling guilty," she says.

Her commitment to exercise, combined with a healthy diet, has paid off: Sarah lost 55 pounds within about a year and she has maintained her weight at a trim and toned 10st 5lb for more than 2 years. She has even won gym-sponsored fitness contests for the most weight lost.

> **WINNING ACTION ➤ ➤ ➤**
>
> **Schedule your exercise as you would a meeting.** If you're busy like Sarah, pencil your exercise on your calendar just like other important things you must do. And don't cancel!

SHE MADE WALKING A SENSORY ADVENTURE

For almost 18 years, Denise Ramirez tried and failed to lose the 80 pounds that stuck around after her pregnancy. She tried exercise classes, but she couldn't stick with the schedule.

"So one day, I put on my headphones and went for a walk," says Denise. "And you know what? I absolutely loved it!"

But hers aren't count-the-minutes-until-you're-done walks where she paces along the same boring route day after day. She ventures into places where she has never been before – new streets, new neighbourhoods, new parks. "Suddenly, I was seeing all of these things that I never knew existed," she says.

For Denise, walking has become a sensory adventure. She's thrilled by the feel of cool morning air, the smell of just-washed laundry hanging out to dry, the sound of lawns being mowed, the sight of frost on grass. "I look for something new every day and file it away in my brain," she says.

She has even made up a game to play along her route. She imagines that she is blind but has been given the gift of sight for one day. So during her walk, she has to soak in everything that she can.

"Open your eyes and be aware," says Denise, who walked off 60 pounds in less than a year. "There is so much out there to see. It's very empowering."

WINNING ACTION ➤➤➤

Head off the beaten path. Denise has the right idea. Walking can get boring if you cover the same route day after day. No matter where you live, you can find new places. For example, check out areas of historical interest, botanical gardens, zoos, tow paths and local parks. Maybe you can't find a new route every day, but take the challenge to come up with 10 different ones. That way, you'll cover the same territory only two or three times a month.

A DOG LED HER TO WEIGHT LOSS

Maureen Keller lost the pounds that marked the end of her old life and the beginning of a new one. And she owes it all to a dog named Bunker.

Recently divorced, Maureen decided to move house to be closer to her family. But she knew it was going to be a long haul, in more ways than one.

During the 6 months leading up to her divorce, Maureen reached a couple of milestones that she found disheartening. First, she turned 50. Second, she climbed four clothing sizes, peaking at 11st 11lb. "Even my 'fat' trousers felt uncomfortable," she recalls.

Overweight and out of shape, Maureen landed in her home town with a purpose but not a plan. Then she met Bunker, a tail-wagging, walk-loving yellow Lab who belonged to her sister, Kathy Irvine and her family.

Just before Maureen's arrival, Kathy and her husband, Dave,

found their workloads growing. The more time they spent at their offices, the less time they had to walk Bunker. His walks were getting shorter and shorter – and he was gaining weight.

"I volunteered to walk Bunker. I love animals and I knew we both needed to slim down," Maureen says. "The first time that we went on a 4-mile route, I was huffing and puffing up the final hill, thinking it would never end. By the end of the walk, Bunker was absolutely exhausted. He slept for the rest of the day."

Their treks soon became a ritual, providing Maureen and Bunker with the exercise they needed. It also gave Maureen time for renewal. Gradually, with less stress and more happiness in her life, she lost 25 pounds. "And Bunker's looking better, too," she adds.

WINNING ACTION ➤ ➤ ➤

Let a dog take you walking. If you have a dog, turn your daily constitutionals into workouts. Walk for 30 to 45 minutes at a comfortably brisk pace – and try not to stop at every tree and lamp post. What if you don't have a dog? Ask a friend or neighbour if you can "borrow" hers. Or volunteer as a dog walker at your local animal shelter. Besides providing exercise, having fun with a dog will change your mindset. How can you focus on problems when you're faced with such a happy, smiling, wagging creature?

SHE SWAM OFF HER POST-RETIREMENT POUNDS

If you need proof that swimming can help you slim down, look no further than Betty Johnson.

All her life, Betty had enjoyed swimming for recreation and physical fitness. While working as an elementary school psychologist, she swam for 45 minutes, twice a week. She rounded out her exercise programme with step-aerobics and strength training.

Shortly after Betty retired, her regular workouts came to a screeching halt. She took time off to decorate her flat and spend 2 months travelling the world. Betty returned home renewed and invigorated – but discouraged about her 15-pound weight gain. She decided to jump back into the pool to work off those extra pounds.

Betty swam for an hour, 3 days a week. She also lifted weights twice a week and enjoyed an occasional bike ride or long walk.

Within 3 months, Betty lost those nagging 15 pounds. She has maintained a healthy weight of 9st 7lb for 6 years.

At 67, Betty remains passionate about swimming. In fact, she even began entering competitions. To date, she has won 11 medals – many for first place – and has advanced to national competition in backstroke and breaststroke.

"Swimming is such a peaceful and relaxing sport," Betty says. "When I do the backstroke, I stare up at the sky and daydream. Runners talk about experiencing a runner's high. After a challenging swim, I enjoy my swimmer's high."

WINNING ACTION ➤ ➤ ➤

Slim down in the swimming pool. You may have heard that swimming isn't an ideal activity for losing weight. But in one study, women who swam burned the same amount of fat as women who walked. The trick is to make sure the water is the right temperature – at least 80°F/28°C. If the water is too cold, you may start feeling hungry as your body craves extra calories to burn for warmth. Also, be sure to swim continuous laps, rather than stopping each time you reach the wall. Do as many laps as you can in 20 to 30 minutes.

SHE FLATTENED HER STOMACH WITH SPINNING

When Mindi Epstein signed up for a Spinning class at a gym near her home, she had no idea that it would be so hard – or that it would change her life so much.

Spinning is road cycling brought indoors. It's done on a specially designed exercise bike and is set to music or a series of visualisations.

"During my first class, I suffered," Mindi, aged 37, laughs. "It was hard work. And the idea of 50 bikes whirring in unison seemed very strange to me." But somewhere near the end of class, Mindi entered what she calls the zone. "The music and energy from the other people took over," she recalls. "I felt so exhilarated that I couldn't wait to come back for more."

After about 3 months of Spinning, Mindi began to notice positive changes in her body. "Trouble spots – your hips, your bottom, your thighs – aren't so much trouble anymore," she says. "In my case, my stomach was always a point of contention. Now, it's flat."

Inspired by her success , Mindi joined a cycling club. These days, she rides three or four times a week, 35 to 80 miles at a time.

Mindi has dropped two dress sizes in 8 months. In return, she has gained a great attitude. "I know that there isn't a hill too steep or a road too long for me to ride," she says. "I'm never so happy as I am when I'm on my bicycle."

WINNING ACTION ➤ ➤ ➤

Get in the "zone". If you're bored by exercise bikes or if you're looking for an indoor alternative to cycling, sign up for a Spinning class. This high-energy activity burns 535 calories in 45 minutes. It also tones abdominal muscles and trims your bottom and thighs. Many gyms and health clubs now offer classes. Check with those in your area.

SHE DANCED HER WAY
TO A PERFECT SIZE 10

When Jennifer Johnson decided to work off her extra pounds, she knew that no ordinary aerobics class would do. She needed an exercise that would be fun. So she signed up for cardio dance lessons at a local gym.

"I've always enjoyed aerobic activities," Jennifer explains. "Between the music and the movement, there's so much energy. When I observed the cardio dance class, I was excited at the prospect of being able to move my body that way."

On her first day, Jennifer felt nothing but frustration. The other students were much more experienced and she questioned whether she'd be able to keep up. But the team atmosphere – everyone working together, like a dance ensemble – soon put her at ease.

Although her only previous experience with dance had been an unpleasant stint as a snowflake in a school production of *The Nutcracker*, Jennifer quickly became a dance enthusiast. She added a class in African dance to her schedule. The more she moved her body, the more it changed shape. "My abdominals have never been as strong as they are now," she enthuses.

The fact that dancing isn't a traditional weight-loss activity isn't lost on Jennifer. She thinks that that's why she enjoys class so much. "Dancing shakes up your routine and stretches you out of your comfort zone," she explains.

When Jennifer started her lessons, she weighed 12st 12lb and wore a size 16-plus. Now, at 37, she's down to 9st 10lb and a size 10 – and she owes it all to dancing. And she can move her body in ways she never imagined. "During the strength and balance exercises at the end of class, we raise one leg straight in front and bring it back around," she says. "I can do that now and I look as good as anyone."

SHE CREDITS HER VICTORY TO YOGA

Melissa MacKinnon overcame a lifelong eating disorder by using the mind/body rituals of yoga to change the way she looked at food and at herself.

Melissa can trace her destructive eating pattern back to the age of 9. "I would starve myself for days before giving in to overwhelming cravings for chocolate biscuits or any other sweets that my mother had on hand," she recalls. "I wasn't too particular, but afterwards, I'd get angry at myself."

It was a vicious cycle that followed her all the way to college. All the while, her weight fluctuated wildly. By the age of 26, she weighed 15st 10lb.

"Intellectually, I knew that I had an eating problem and that it was only making my life worse," Melissa says. "But my mind and body were at absolute odds and I couldn't get them to reconcile."

Until she discovered yoga.

"It looked so relaxing and easy, so perfect for my imperfect body," Melissa says. And she knew that she had to get active if she wanted to slim down. She had tried aerobics, but it just didn't appeal to her.

Yoga did more than get Melissa in shape. It had positive effects that she never expected. Her energy level soared. As she became more attuned to her body, she understood its need for proper nourishment. She craved greens and vegetables instead of chocolate. She replaced refined sugars with brown-rice syrup. "As yoga rewired my mind, I learned to take better care of my body," she says.

In 8 months, Melissa lost 60 pounds. Now, at 33, she has maintained her weight for 7 years without resorting to the extremes of bingeing and starving that once tore her life apart. "And I owe it all to yoga," she says.

In fact, she's so thankful to yoga for changing her life that she qualified as an instructor in order to share its benefits with others.

WINNING ACTION ➤ ➤ ➤

Trim and tone your body with yoga. Gentle and low-impact, yoga may not seem like a calorie-burning activity, but it is. And it has other benefits as well. As Melissa discovered, the discipline of yoga has a mind-body effect that can go a long way towards untying some of the mental knots that may be standing between you and your weight-loss goals.

FENCING BROKE DOWN HIS FITNESS BARRIER

At the tender age of 21, Dan Collins was so overweight and out of shape that his doctor feared he was killing himself.

"I was 5 foot 10½ inches and weighed 17st 1lb," he says. "I was diagnosed with high blood pressure and my doctor was concerned enough to put me on medication."

That was in 1984. Rather than sit back and let medications take control of his life, the young newspaper reporter embarked on a complete body makeover. He cut down on the salt in his diet, put the brakes on his runaway eating habits and began walking and using an exercise bike regularly.

Two years later, Dan had his blood pressure under control and was down to a lean 13 stone. He felt and looked great but was afraid that he was entering an exercise slump. "I didn't mind the walking and other exercises, but I really wanted a different kind of sport that I could really get into," he says. "I knew that was important if I was going to keep the weight off for good."

For Dan, that sport was fencing. It piqued his interest because it is both physically and mentally demanding. Working up a sweat was fun and exciting each time he picked up his foil and donned his mask. "People don't realise that a good fencer needs both aerobic and anaerobic conditioning as well as a sense of strategy and emotional control," says Dan, now the co-founder of a fencing club.

Dan still fences every week, just like he's been doing for the last 14 years. He also works out at home using an exercise bike and free weights to enhance his fencing performance. After all these years, it's safe to say that this lean, mean fencing machine has found the perfect activity to help him keep the weight off.

WINNING ACTION ➤ ➤ ➤

Go for the unusual and exotic. Learning how to move your body – and enjoy it – is personal. If you are having a hard time sticking with a particular workout regime, try something unusual or unconventional, like African dance, tai chi or scuba-diving. Part of the journey of weight loss is discovering and uncovering the real you. Let your workouts be an expression of your inner self. If not now, when? Enjoy today!

HE PICKED UP A RACKET – AND ACED WEIGHT LOSS

Murray Hann admits that he wasn't the kind of person that you'd expect to find on a tennis court. At 22st 7lb, he looked more like a spectator than a player. "But I played a decent game, even as a fat guy," he says.

His love of the sport helped him launch a regular fitness programme – and helped him lose almost half of his body weight.

Murray, a 38-year-old mechanical engineer had a weight problem throughout his entire life. "I grew up with a wonderful mother who regularly baked biscuits for my brother and me," he recalls. "I ate more than I should have and it showed."

At 30, Murray started feeling self-conscious about his size. "I didn't want to spend the rest of my life alone and I believed that that's what would happen if I didn't slim down," he says. "No woman on Earth would be tolerant enough to see through all that fat."

As much as he wanted to shed the extra pounds, Murray refused to go on a diet. "Diets provide only temporary results," he explains. "I wanted to lose the weight permanently. I knew that that would mean making lifestyle changes."

Murray thought about how much he enjoyed tennis, and a number of other sports. He figured that he could stick with a regular exercise programme, which in turn would help him lose weight.

"I made up my mind to work out every day, no matter what," he says. "Sometimes, I felt selfish because I put exercise so high on my priority list. It became almost as important to me as food, water and sleep."

His brother gave him a rowing machine, which Murray used every night. "I wouldn't fix dinner until I completed 40 minutes," he says. He continued to play an occasional game of tennis. As his fitness improved, he graduated to squash, then mountain biking, then walking, then jogging, then running.

To support his new exercise habit, Murray began paying more attention to his food choices. He cut back on fat while making sure to get an adequate amount of protein.

With regular workouts and a better diet, Murray was able to take off 150 pounds in about a year. He has maintained his weight at 11st 11lb since 1992.

Exercise had another, unexpected benefit that made Murray even happier than his trim physique. He met his wife, Susan, on the squash courts at a local leisure centre. "We played against each other and she kicked my butt," he recalls.

These days, Murray and Susan often work out together as part of their active lifestyle. In addition, during his lunch hour, Murray usually runs with a group of colleagues. "I enjoy the sunshine, fresh air and camaraderie more than food," he says.

WINNING ACTION ➤➤➤

Do what you love; love what you do. There's no rule saying that you have to walk or run or pedal a bike to lose weight. Anything that gets your body moving burns calories. So find an activity that you love. Murray is a great role model: he loves tennis and he used it as a springboard to establishing a regular exercise programme. The point is that if you enjoy what you're doing, you're more likely to do it.

ADVENTURE LED TO A NEW LIFE AND A NEW WAISTLINE

What do maps, compasses and insect repellent have to do with weight loss? If you're Sharon Evans, a 38-year-old accountant, the answer would have to be "everything." Back in 1992, Sharon took up orienteering and finally shed the 20 extra pounds that she had been carrying on her 5-foot-5-inch frame.

Orienteering is a cross-country sport where people find their way through unfamiliar terrain using only a compass and a map. Sharon got involved as a way to improve her skills in another sport – backpacking. "I'm what you might call geographically challenged," she explains. "I wanted to learn how to use a compass when I blaze trails."

So when Sharon joined her local orienteering club, weight loss wasn't even on her mind. But it turned out to be a fabulous perk. Instead of spending time munching on junk food in front of the TV, she was out in the fresh air learning navigational skills that called on her mental and physical faculties. Better fitness would contribute to better competition times, so Sharon finally had a reason to stick with a jogging programme. Her club's social network gave her support not only as her orienteering skills grew but as her waistline shrank. "They were all so excited to share their experiences; it was very contagious and inspiring," she says.

Today, Sharon is a seasoned orienteering veteran. Moreover, she has maintained her fit form and taken on other outdoor challenges. "Through the skills I've learned in orienteering, plus the better fitness level I'm at, I feel more confident to do things like backpacking, climbing, even working on a horse farm," she says. She's even training to be a volunteer firefighter.

For Sharon, navigating her way to successful weight loss has been a life-enhancing experience.

WINNING ACTION ➤ ➤ ➤

Find an activity that suits your personality. Weight loss can happen with no effort at all if you can make fitness a hobby, as Sharon did. You don't have to take up orienteering or rock climbing. Any activity that involves a social network can make getting fit a lot of fun.

LITTLE TRICKS LED TO LASTING SUCCESS

Ileen Kaplan carried around an unwanted 10 pounds for years until she started practising one weight-loss tip that we've all been hearing for years: take the stairs instead of the lift.

She's living proof that it works. "I tried everything to get rid of those 10 pounds," said Ileen, 49. "I ate low-fat snacks. I worked out. I lost weight, but it always came back." Then, after reading how small lifestyle changes can produce big results, she decided to find out if little things really do count.

"I started parking the car at the far end of the car park instead of in the closest spot," she says. "I used the stairs instead of lifts. I made two trips carrying the groceries instead of one."

She didn't even notice what was happening until her clothes got so loose she stepped onto the scales. "I couldn't believe it – those 10 pounds were finally gone," she says. That was more than 3 years ago. The weight has stayed off ever since.

She still works out and eats healthily. The key to keeping off extra pounds, she says, is to take extra steps whenever possible.

"I shifted my attention from thinking about what I should or shouldn't eat to thinking about how great I feel when I move my body," Ileen says. "Now I see even the littlest things, like walking a quarter-mile to the supermarket, as opportunities, because they feel so good."

WINNING ACTION ➤ ➤ ➤

Let your feet help you achieve your goal weight. Look for opportunities to incorporate extra steps into your routine. If you're expecting a lengthy phone call, take the call on a cordless phone and walk around while talking. If you take a bus, get off a stop or two early and walk the rest. The possibilities are endless.

SHE GOT IN TOUCH
WITH HER THINNER CHILD

Many of us talk about recapturing our youth. Kirie Pedersen actually did it. And it helped her get rid of 40 unwanted pounds at the same time.

Kirie, a 48-year-old freelance writer, prided herself on leading a healthy lifestyle. Her diet consisted primarily of grains and vegetables – little meat, little sugar, no junk food. And she walked for a half-hour to an hour every day.

So when the scales showed that her weight had crept up to 11st 5lb, Kirie could come up with only one explanation. "Almost every day for 6 years, my job had me sitting for 8 to 9 hours at a stretch," she says. "Even though I was eating well and exercising regularly, most of the time I was glued to a chair."

Kirie became convinced that if she could reclaim some of the nervous energy that she had as a child, she could burn a few more calories over the course of a day. So she found ways to incorporate playful, childlike movements into her life.

Every morning, she woke with a big stretch. She swung her arms vigorously when she walked. "I'd act childishly in the privacy of my home office," she says. "I'd set a timer to go off every hour. That was my cue to get up and move. For 15 minutes, I'd squat, skip, wiggle, dance, whatever I felt like doing."

One year after she began incorporating childlike movements into her daily routine, Kirie went shopping for clothes with her daughter. "I was comfortable with my wardrobe of baggy clothes, but my daughter persuaded me to try on a pair of jeans, something that I don't usually wear," Kirie recalls. "I figured that I'd need a size 14 or 16. My daughter looked at me and said, 'I don't think you realise how much weight you've lost!'"

Her daughter was right. Kirie had taken off 40 pounds – and slimmed down to a size 8 – simply by acting like a child again.

SHE LOST WEIGHT BY ACCIDENT

Having discovered the secret of calorie-burning chores, Kay Black has never had a trimmer figure – or a cleaner, more organised house.

When Kay, 55, recalls how she started losing weight, she laughs, "It was an accident." Not that she didn't *want* to lose weight. Sure, she was carrying an unwanted 60 pounds on her frame; and of course she was tired of being mistaken for her daughter's grandmother. But she simply couldn't find the motivation to exercise.

Then Kay decided to organise her family's books – all 5,400 of them – by cataloguing them on her new computer. "I teach college geography, so I do a lot of reading," she explains. "Besides, my family just loves books." Each night, she'd carry several armloads upstairs, type up the data and take the books back downstairs. She'd stretch for 15 to 20 minutes to prevent next-day stiffness, then take a hot bath. By the time the project was complete, she had lost 5 pounds!

Kay decided that this was too easy not to continue. "Nothing breeds success like success," she says. She stripped and repainted her daughter's room and rearranged the attic. She shovelled snow in the winter and turned her garden into a "gym" in the summer. She took up walking, too, usually getting a 40- to 50-minute workout 5 days a week.

These days, Kay is a svelte 8 stone, down from her heaviest of 12st 4lb. Her family's book collection is as organised as ever. And her house is so tidy that she's even prepared for unexpected guests.

WINNING ACTION ➤ ➤ ➤

Turn housework into weight loss. Not interested in walking, running or swimming laps? Then don't! There are plenty of tasks around your home that can help you slim down. Here's a rundown of the calorie-burning potential of some common household chores. (The numbers were tabulated for 1 hour of activity by a 150-pound person.)

Scrubbing the floor	374
Painting the exterior of the house	340
Gardening	340
Mowing the lawn	306

GRANDMA LOSES 50 BY KEEPING STEP WITH A CHILD

Dolly Higgin's slow-speed life – and her metabolism – cranked up several notches once she started chasing Alisha.

When 70-year-old Dolly retired, her lifestyle took a turn for the worse. The grandmother found herself sleeping and eating a lot. Soon, she weighed 12st 2lb, far too much for her 5-foot-2-inch frame. The excess weight pressed on a herniated disc in her back, leaving her bed bound for weeks. Then she found out that she had high blood pressure and borderline diabetes.

Dolly knew that her weight had contributed to her health

problems. She also knew that she needed to dump those excess pounds. But she couldn't get herself started. A favour for her daughter turned out to be the boost she needed.

"My daughter had taken a third job and needed me to help watch Alisha, my granddaughter," Dolly explains. "I was thrilled. I needed a reason to get out of bed every morning."

On fair-weather days, Dolly walked Alisha to school in the morning, then returned to pick her up in the afternoon. When Dolly took Alisha to the local pool twice a week, she did some swimming herself. She also started swimming on "senior days". As Alisha got older, Dolly joined her for bike rides, an activity she enjoyed so much that she even bought an exercise bike for winter.

During the first year and a half, Dolly lost 40 pounds, going from size 20 to 12. Today, she feels great and has an excellent health record. Though she no longer watches her granddaughter as often, Dolly has maintained her new, active lifestyle.

MOTHER NATURE GOT HIM IN SHAPE

John Bradley always loved being outdoors. As a youngster, he spent many more summer nights sleeping outside than in. His days were filled with work on his family's potato farm, fishing, swimming, canoeing and hiking in the woods.

Now aged 45, John still finds joy in the great outdoors. It not only relaxes him but it also helped him lose 30 pounds.

John, who ran his own farm for more than 20 years before becoming a university student had a weight problem for most of his life. He ate too much of the wrong kinds of foods and despite his active lifestyle, it showed.

"My family always kept a lot of sweets around the house," he says. "And I had a special fondness for chips and Coke. I drank Coke all the time."

Every now and then, John would diet and lose some weight, only to regain it. By 40, he reached 15st 10lb. "I realised that slimming down wouldn't get any easier as I got older," he says. "And I knew that I'd be a lot healthier without the extra pounds. So I made up my mind to get rid of them for good."

John paid more attention to his food intake, eliminating fried foods, desserts and high-calorie snacks. He kept an eye on his portion sizes, too. For exercise, he began doing situps, working up to 100, five times per week. But what really made a difference, he says, were his nightly nature walks.

Every evening after dinner, John, sometimes accompanied by his wife, would go for a walk on his 270-acre farm. He'd wander for an hour, sometimes two, observing nature in all her glory.

John so enjoyed his nature walks that he never really thought of them as exercise. Yet in combination with his improved eating habits and his situp regime, they got him down to a healthy 13st 8lb in about 6 months. He's been holding steady since 1996.

"If I wasn't active, I'd gain weight quickly," John says. "But the exercise that I do is a pleasure. I'm always glad to get outdoors. It's where I feel best. It's the place where I most love to be."

HE DROPPED 200 GETTING LOST IN THOUGHT

Seven years ago, Mitch Lipka tipped the scales at 32st 2lb, thanks in large part to a steady diet of high-fat foods. But he never got serious about slimming down until the day he tried to climb a short flight of stairs to his mother's flat. The effort left Mitch, who could no longer fit through a turnstile or use a normal dining chair, exhausted and gasping for air. On the spot, he resolved to lose weight.

He started by giving up meats and fried foods, then eliminated cheese, ice cream and other high-fat fare. In their place, he learned to prepare low-fat meals, using a cookbook that his mother gave him. The pounds started coming off almost immediately.

Inspired by his progress, Mitch started plotting his next strategy: exercise. At first, he tried walking around the block. But because his job as a newspaper reporter had him working odd hours, he had to find an activity that fitted better into his busy schedule. So he invested in an exercise bike, which he rode when he got home from work. "I'd set little goals for myself," he recalls. "I'd ride for 5 minutes the first five sessions, then 7 minutes the next five sessions and so on."

Of course, some nights Mitch could hardly bear to look at his bike, much less ride it. That's when his diversionary tactic came into play. He'd throw a towel or a T-shirt over the timer, then concentrate on something else. He'd get so lost in thought that before he knew it, his time was up.

After 2 years of his diet-and-exercise regime, Mitch had lost 200 pounds. Five years later, at 34, he's still fit and feeling good about himself.

WINNING ACTION ➤ ➤ ➤

Let your imagination go. Boredom can wreck even the best-laid exercise plans. If you're not enjoying what you're doing, chances are, you won't stick with it. So find ways to make your workout interesting. Mitch hides the timer and thinks about something else. If you're using a exercise bike or other fitness equipment, try watching TV, flicking through a magazine or cranking up some Tina Turner, Madonna or your favourite up-tempo tunes. Personally, as dull as it seems, I'm a fan of nothingness, like Mitch. I like quiet time when I'm on my treadmill. My mind wanders everywhere!

VARIETY SPICES
UP HER WORKOUTS

Whenever Cheryl Allard goes to the gym, she abides by her 10-minute rule: use one machine for 10 minutes, then move on to something else. This strategy helped her beat the boredom that nearly ended her exercise programme. It also helped her lose 100 pounds.

Cheryl began working out in 1997 after finding out that she had high blood pressure. At the time, she weighed 18st 4lb. "I was chubby even as a child," recalls the 50-year-old sewing machine consultant. "Living through World War II, when food was rationed, my parents had the mindset that food was never to be wasted. I was raised to clean my plate."

As Cheryl got older, the pounds kept piling on. "I tried every diet under the sun to slim down," she says. "Once, I even lost 40 pounds, but they all came back."

Then, Cheryl's husband persuaded her to get a physical. "I hadn't been to our family doctor in years and my husband kept bugging me to go," she explains. "I went just to keep him quiet."

But Cheryl was the one left speechless after her doctor handed her a prescription for blood pressure medication. "That got me motivated to lose," she says. "I didn't want to be taking pills for the rest of my life."

Cheryl went to a nutritional consultant, who helped her revamp her eating habits. She also joined a local gym, where she started using the aerobic-exercise equipment. "I felt self-conscious at first because of my size," she says.

Over time, her self-confidence grew – as did her boredom. Even though she varied her workouts, they seemed to drag on and on. But she knew that she couldn't stop exercising.

So she decided to add some variety to her workout routine. Rather than spending all of her time on one piece of equipment, she'd stay on for just 10 minutes, then switch. "I can do anything for 10 minutes," she says. "Even though I detest riding that bike, I do it, knowing that it's only going to be for 10 minutes." Usually, she ends up using four or five different machines.

That did the trick. Cheryl found herself looking forward to her workouts so much that she started going to the gym 6 days a week. Within a year of launching her weight-loss programme, she took off 100 pounds.

In the years since, Cheryl has continued to eat sensibly and exercise regularly. And it shows: her weight has held steady at 11st 11lb. Even better, her blood pressure has returned to a healthy level and she was able to stop taking her medication.

"When my son got married not too long ago, my relatives flew in from abroad," she says. "They were commenting on how much weight I had lost and how good I look. More important to me, though, is that I feel great!"

FRIENDS HELP FRIENDS LOSE

In 1994, Anita Beattie's doctor gave her a harsh ultimatum: "Lose weight or don't come back to see me, because you're wasting my time and yours."

His words stung, but Anita knew that her doctor was right. She weighed 11st 3lb and she also had diabetes – a bad combination, to say the least. "He kicked me where it hurts and that's what I needed," says the 67 year old.

Determined to get in shape, Anita immediately enrolled in a 4-day hospital weight-loss programme, where she learned the importance of eating better and exercising more. She began applying her new nutrition knowledge immediately, making healthier food choices and controlling her portion sizes.

For exercise, Anita decided to try walking. But she knew that she'd need support – someone to push her through the front door when she felt like staying at home. So she recruited some friends to join her. "Most of them are about my age and like me, they want to exercise to keep themselves fit and healthy," she says.

Anita and her exercise buddies have established a daily routine. They choose a time and place to meet, then set out for a brisk 3-mile walk. For Anita, knowing that people are counting on her helps her shake off thoughts of skipping her workout. "Maybe it's a little cold or maybe I just don't feel like walking," she says. "I think of my friends waiting for me and I don't want to leave them stranded."

When Anita goes to Florida for the winter, she doesn't leave her workout behind. She has exercise buddies there, too. Every day, they meet at 9 o'clock in the morning for a walk up and down the beach.

Anita's buddy-system approach to exercise helped her take off 38 pounds, which she has kept off for 6 years. And with her doctor's guidance, she was able to taper off the insulin that she used to control her diabetes.

WINNING ACTION ➤ ➤ ➤

Do walking workouts with a friend. In one survey, women cited having an exercise buddy as one of the main reasons they were able to stick with a fitness programme. Finding an exercise buddy has several advantages. You develop a sense of obligation to the other person, so you're less likely to skip a workout. You motivate one another and maybe engage in a bit of friendly competition. And you're safer when you're with someone than when you're alone.

THEY'RE COMMITTED TO EACH OTHER – AND TO HEALTHY LIVING

Talk about your dynamic duo!

In the mid-1990s, Patti Pottebaum and her husband, Gary,

kicked their 20-year smoking habits. The couple say that attacking the problem as a team helped them succeed.

But in the months that followed, the usually trim Patti and Gary found their waistlines expanding – a byproduct, they believe, of substituting snacks for smoking. In 2 years, they wound up gaining 48 pounds between them.

So, in January 1997, 41-year-old Patti and 44-year-old Gary decided to slim down. "We were tired of having to loosen our belts and buy bigger clothing," Patti explains. "Plus, we were beginning to experience some post-40 aches and pains. We just didn't feel like ourselves."

Because the team approach had worked so well when they quit smoking, Patti and Gary decided to use it again to lose weight. They agreed to cook and eat low-fat meals loaded with fruits and vegetables; red meats and fried foods were to be used only sparingly.

Although they initially exercised separately – she with step-aerobics classes, he with running – workouts became a team effort before long. "We have always been a couple who enjoys doing things together, so we started walking in the mornings before work," Patti says. "I had an easier time staying motivated when I knew that I'd be exercising with Gary." They even kept things interesting by playing golf together and placing friendly wagers on each round.

Neither Pottebaum wants to let the other down by missing a workout. For example, since Gary is more lively in the mornings, his get-up-and-go helps Patti get out of bed, even if she says that she's not in the mood for walking. Their commitment to wellness and to each other resulted in Patti losing 25 pounds and Gary losing 23 in a little more than 9 months.

Now that they are back to their trim sizes – she a 12 or 14, he a 36-inch waist – the Pottebaums have no intention of falling out of shape. "I like being in good shape and I feel so much better," Gary says. "We want to stay active and healthy forever so we can enjoy the rest of our lives to the fullest."

SHE FOUND HER
MOTIVATION IN CYBERSPACE

Stephanie Caviness wanted to slim down. But the 33-year-old had a hard time sticking with an exercise routine. So she turned to her computer for help and she ended up losing 23 pounds.

For Stephanie, exercise was nothing new. She had tried several times in the past to get in shape. "I had been gaining weight ever since I was in college," she recalls. "I wanted to look better and feel better. But every time I started an exercise programme, I'd lose interest. Eventually, I'd abandon my workouts."

By 1998, Stephanie weighed 12st 5lb. "I'm 5 foot 9 inches, so I wasn't really obese," she says. "But I was having problems with my heart – it raced and sometimes skipped beats. My doctor attributed those irregularities to the fact that I was in such poor condition aerobically."

At last, Stephanie found her motivation to lose weight and get fit. She pursued a variety of activities – step aerobics, aqua-aerobics, running, even salsa dancing. She made some dietary changes, too, eating more fruits and vegetables, watching her fat intake, measuring portions and drinking lots of water.

Her efforts paid off: her heart health improved and as a

bonus, her body looked trimmed and toned. She marvelled at how the pounds disappeared so quickly, but worried about whether she could continue losing. More and more, exercise seemed like a chore. "Even though I was doing a lot of different things, I felt myself losing interest," she says. "But I didn't want to sabotage the progress that I had made."

Convinced that others must be facing the same problem, Stephanie pondered the idea of forming an exercise support group. "There's strength in numbers," she says. "Staying motivated is a lot easier when you're working with a group rather than on your own."

Stephanie decided to post a message on Diet Talk, a website that she had been frequenting for information and support since starting her weight-loss programme. "I had got to know a number of people through the message boards and chat rooms and I suspected that some of them were struggling with exercise, as I was," she explains. She was right: about 15 people responded to her message.

In January 1999, Stephanie and her online buddies kicked off their Exercise Challenge. Each person has a goal of exercising at least five times a week. "Everyone's workout is a little different, based on individual abilities and objectives," Stephanie explains. "That doesn't matter, as long as we're doing something." The group members e-mail Stephanie at least every 3 days and often daily, to report on their activities. Stephanie posts the results online on a monthly basis.

"Every month, 80 to 90 per cent of us meet the challenge," she says. "That's been really encouraging."

Even more encouraging is the support that participants give one another. "The group changes in size from month to month, from the core membership of 15 to as many as 40," Stephanie says. "We've become almost like a family. We talk about our weight struggles, but we talk about other areas of our lives as well. And when one of us succeeds, all of us succeed."

HIS NICKNAME STILL STICKS

During college, Robert Kilroy was so tall and thin – 6 foot tall and 11st 6lb – that his friends called him Stick. But within a few years of graduation, he literally outgrew his nickname. Stick was stuck at 14st 4lb.

As a naval flight officer, Robert bounced from one military base to another, spending between 3 and 6 months in places as far-flung as Alaska and Japan. "We'd fly for 12 hours a day and by the time we'd get back to base, the restaurants would be closed," he recalls. "I'd eat whatever I had stashed in my room. And it was usually junk." His hectic schedule made a regular exercise routine difficult, too.

In 1996, Robert left the Navy to study law. Every day, on his drive between home and college, he'd pass a gym. Eventually, he decided to join. "I didn't like the way I felt or looked," he says. "I had to get back to a weight that I was comfortable with." He made a promise to himself to work out 5 days a week, whether on his way to school or on his way home. Since he didn't have to drive out of his way, he had no excuse for not exercising.

This strategy worked so well that Robert, now aged 35, was able to take off 23 pounds. And when he relocated in 1998, he made sure to join a gym that was located along his commuting route.

"I go almost every day on my way home from work," he says. "Sometimes I play basketball, sometimes I ride an exercise bike. Best of all, I've maintained my weight."

WINNING ACTION ➤➤➤

Find a gym that's on your way. With a gym, as with any property, the important thing is location, location, location. If you have to drive 30 minutes across town to work out, chances are, you won't do it. Follow Robert's lead and look for a gym somewhere along your route to and from work. If you pass by the place every day, you'll be more likely to go.

OPRAH MADE HER MOVE HER MUSCLES

Nica Russell was certain that she'd never get out of the negative mindset that allowed her weight to escalate to 19st 4lb. Then she saw a talk show that completely changed her life.

"Television programmes and commercials about weight loss would bring me to tears, but they couldn't inspire me to get off the sofa and *do* something," says 36-year-old Nica. "Then I happened to catch an Oprah Winfrey show in which Oprah was crying and talking about her lifelong struggle with her weight. I felt that she was talking directly to me, that she knew exactly how I was feeling. She motivated me to tackle my weight problem."

The next day, Nica went to the nearest shopping centre and headed straight for the video shop. She scanned the rows of aerobic exercise videos and purchased a selection of tapes with workouts ranging from beginner to advanced. Every day for 4 months, in the privacy of her own home, she did a 45-minute video workout. "At first, I could do only about 1 per cent of the routines. I felt like I was going to die," she says. "But every time I thought about giving up, I remembered Oprah's words. I found myself going longer without a break and without feeling like passing out. Eventually, I could do my tape routines from beginning to end." At that point, she felt confident enough to visit a gym.

With guidance from a personal trainer, Nica started lifting weights. Over time, she became an exercise fanatic, working out for 3 hours a day, 7 days a week. "I was obsessed," she says, "but I had a goal to meet." To help her get there, she made some adjustments in her eating habits, giving up fried foods and filling up on fruits and vegetables. Within 7 months, she lost 135 pounds.

Satisfied with her new, slim physique, Nica began having second thoughts about going to the gym. She was tired of paying the high membership fee, fighting traffic to get there and queuing for equipment. So she decided to create a gym at home.

Over a 2-year period, Nina invested in advanced aerobic exercise videos, sets of 5- to 25-pound dumbbells and weight-training equipment with a step attachment. "My home gym definitely motivates me to stay fit," she says. "Without it, I wouldn't work out as consistently or maintain my weight."

Today, Nica works out for an hour, 4 or 5 days a week. She has maintained her weight at a healthy 9st 9lb for 4 years.

WINNING ACTION ➤ ➤ ➤

Build your own gym. If you're not comfortable going to the gym, invest in some exercise equipment for your home. Start by purchasing aerobic exercise videos or a treadmill for walking or running. Then work your way up to dumbbells and weight-training equipment. You'll have all the essentials you need to stay fit, without the inconvenience of packing a bag, jumping in your car and driving to the gym. I invested in a treadmill and I love it.

A FRIENDLY NUDGE
GAVE HER STRENGTH

When Lynn Oatman sits down in her swivel rocking chair to watch television after a long day of work, she doesn't stop moving.

Instead, the 48-year-old picks up a pair of 3-pound hand weights and starts pumping. For about a half-hour during her TV time each night, she hoists the weights up and down behind her head to exercise her triceps, then curls them forwards towards her chest to work her biceps. Because she has filled her days with healthy lifestyle choices like this, Lynn has shed 60 pounds in 2 years, dropping from a size 26 to a size 16.

Back when Lynn weighed about 17st 2lb, she was growing frustrated over her failed attempts to slim down. One evening over dinner, two friends told her that they'd noticed her unhappiness. Along with their candid observation, they gave her a 10-week membership in a weight-loss group. It helped spark a change in her life.

Through the weight-loss group, Lynn learned how to eat more healthily. Her portion sizes got smaller and her food choices shifted towards fruits, vegetables and whole grains. "But I don't exclude any foods," she says. "That only leads to bingeing."

For exercise, Lynn joined a fitness programme sponsored by the university where she worked. The programme's instructors advised Lynn to start doing aerobic exercise. Now each morning, before she heads to her job as a secretary in the university's law department, she works out for 1 hour and 15 minutes in the university's gym. Most of her time is spent on a rowing machine and elliptical stepper, though she lifts weights, too.

"I've gone from somebody who could barely lift a 10-pound bag of potatoes to somebody who can bench-press 75 pounds five times," she says. "It makes me feel powerful and it's the first time in my life that I've really felt physically powerful."

> ### WINNING ACTION ➤ ➤ ➤
>
> *Turn your armchair into a workout space.* Keep a pair of small hand weights near the chair, sofa or other spot where you relax in the evening. As you unwind from your day, you can squeeze in more exercise while in a comfortable place. And keeping the weights there will serve as a reminder of your new, healthy lifestyle.

WHEN IT COMES TO EXERCISE, THE SKY'S THE LIMIT

For most people, holidays and plane travel are times to sit back and relax. For 48-year-old Kathleen Rayson of Munich, Germany, they're a signal to start moving.

Kathleen, her husband, Tom and their son, T. J., journey to Florida twice a year to spend time at their second home in Sarasota. In the past, Kathleen barely moved on the 9½-hour flight from Germany to Florida and she consumed anything that the airline attendants offered her, because there was nothing else to do.

To make matters worse, Kathleen's activity level didn't improve much when she touched down. "I didn't do any formal exercise in Germany, but I was up and down the four floors of my house dozens of times a day and I always cycled to the food shops," she says. "In Florida, I sat in a ranch house and drove everywhere."

Kathleen suspects that all the inactivity pushed her weight upwards. "Of course, when I was back home in Germany, all that high-fat German food didn't help much – nor did the German beer," she says.

By January 1998, she reached her top weight of 13st 2lb. "I had kind of been accepting my weight gain, but what those scales said was really a shock," Kathleen recalls.

Trying to slim down in a country that's known for its sausages and potatoes was, to say the least, a challenge. But Kathleen worked on reducing her fat intake and eating more whole grains, fruits and vegetables. For exercise, she joined a fitness club where one of the personal trainers customised a workout regime for her that included toning and cardiovascular routines. She also attended aerobics classes. By the time she arrived in the United States that summer, she was down 22 pounds.

She didn't want to lose ground by being idle in Sarasota. "Instead of sitting around all day, my husband and I walked every morning for an hour, then used free weights and did situps for another half-hour," she says. "The activity curbed my desire to eat."

On the flight back to Germany, instead of just sitting, Kathleen got up and exercised six times. She went into the galley and did deep knee bends and ran in place. She also walked laps around the big 747. She repeated the routine about every hour. "I didn't gain a pound that trip," she says. "And what a great way to beat the boredom!"

Now 40 pounds lighter, Kathleen takes her walking shorts with her wherever she goes, even if it's a weekend trip to London to visit relatives. And she always stands up and moves around the plane. It not only prevents boredom and improves her circulation, it stops her from eating.

WINNING ACTION ▶▶▶

Travelling? Take your workout with you. I've learned that exercise doesn't have to take a holiday. Pack a pair of comfortable walking shoes and take a brisk walk every day. I've found that going for an early-morning walk in a new city is the best way to really get to know it and feel like you're actually there, even if you're on a business trip. On long flights, walk around the plane cabin and stretch.

NO MORE WINTER FAT

Karen Uhlenhuth never needed a calendar to know what month it was. She could tell by the number on her scales.

"It never failed," says the 42-year-old writer. "In mid to late November, I'd start gaining – usually about 10 pounds, 15 at the most. Then in April, I'd start losing."

While Karen came to expect these seasonal ups and downs, she didn't welcome them. Eventually, she made up her mind that they had to stop.

"It was autumn 1996," she recalls. "Winter was approaching and I could feel the pounds creeping on again. I started thinking about how I never felt as well in the winter as I did in the summer and I blamed the extra weight." On the spot, she resolved to maintain her "summer weight" – 10st 2lb on her 5-foot-8½-inch frame – throughout the year.

A vegetarian and healthy eater, Karen knew her problem was her activity level. "I'm a compulsive gardener," she says. "In spring and summer, I'd work outside until nightfall. But I couldn't do that in autumn and winter." Likewise, she'd run 5 miles two or three times a week in nice weather. But once the temperatures dropped, she'd pack up her running shoes.

Karen realised that she had to stay active all year-round. So she began changing activities with the seasons. When the weather put an end to gardening and running outdoors, she moved her exercise indoors, swimming at the local leisure centre and working out on a cross-training machine at home. "It took some effort on my part," she says. "There were days when I got home from work and all I wanted to do was eat dinner and lie on the sofa. But I'd remind myself that if I didn't want to gain weight, I had to *move*."

For Karen, staying active all year round made all the difference. She hasn't noticed any seasonal fluctuations in her weight since 1996, when she launched her autumn and winter fitness programme. To this day, she maintains her weight at a healthy 10st 2lb.

"I try to stay active, even though it's much harder during the winter," Karen says. "I just tell myself that as soon as spring comes around, I'll be outdoors, doing all of the activities that I love."

WINNING ACTION ➤➤➤

Keep moving, no matter what the season. It's a fact that we humans tend to be less active during the autumn and winter months, when the temperature drops and the weather turns nasty. Just like bears, we want to hibernate. Don't let your fitness programme falter at this time of year. Invest in some home exercise equipment or join a health club. If there's a college in your area, find out whether its gym facilities are open to the public. Or take up an outdoor activity such as skiing, ice-skating or running, all of which are wonderful winter fat-and-calorie burners.

SHE SLIMMED DOWN ON THE PATH TO SELF-DISCOVERY

In 1996, when Linda Christopher began walking during her lunch hour, she didn't foresee the profound impact that it would have on her life. Sure, she lost weight – her real purpose from the start. But along the way, she reconnected with nature, reaffirmed her faith in God and rediscovered herself.

Back then, Linda was grappling with a lifelong weight problem that seemed to grow worse as she got older. She was fed up with dieting and with losing and regaining the same pounds. "I stopped weighing myself when I hit 13st 2lb," says the 41-year-old teacher. "But I know that I got even heavier, because I could barely fit into my size-20 clothes."

Her too-small wardrobe only reinforced Linda's dissatisfaction with how she looked and felt. It gave her the incentive to make some positive changes in her life.

"I just reached a point where I couldn't handle it anymore," she continues. "Instead of dwelling on weight loss, I shifted my focus to a healthier lifestyle."

With that goal clear in her mind, Linda began to improve her eating habits. She tried hard to rein in her stress-induced binges. And if she felt that she had to eat something, she chose crunchy carrots or an apple instead of biscuits or crisps.

For exercise, she swam a couple of times of week at a local pool. And every day on her lunch break, she took a 20-minute walk through a nearby park. Those walks evolved into mini-spiritual journeys as Linda found herself using the time to commune with nature. "I had always enjoyed being outside, but between work and other activities, I had got away from it," she explains. "Those lunchtime walks helped me rediscover my love of the outdoors. There were so many sights and sounds and smells that I had forgotten."

Amid all of that natural splendour, Linda experienced a sort of spiritual reawakening. Her faith in God deepened and she felt more at peace with herself. "Walking was as good for my mind and spirit as for my body," she says. "I felt so much better and in ways that I never expected."

Linda came to treasure her lunchtime walks so much that they gradually stretched from 20 minutes to an hour. Within 6 months, she lost more than 30 pounds. Out went those size 20s, replaced with size 14s.

Linda has maintained her weight at a healthy 11 stone ever since. She has become such an avid outdoorswoman that she leads hikes for her local fitness group. Every Sunday morning, she spends at least an hour wandering the woods near her home –

reconnecting with nature, with God and with herself.

"I feel much better physically – and as a bonus, I've got back in touch with my spirituality," she says. "That has made all the difference in my health and my life."

WINNING ACTION ➤ ➤ ➤

Transform your walk into a moving meditation. Walking is a wonderfully simple exercise for losing weight and getting fit. With its rhythmic pace, it can become meditative, especially when you're alone. Use that time for personal reflection and renewal. It not only makes your workout go faster but it also mentally and spiritually rejuvenates you.

HE RAN AWAY
FROM A WEIGHT PROBLEM

As a child, Robert Kim used food as a security blanket, a means of coping with a stressful home environment. Then, 16 years ago, he put down his fork and picked up a pair of running shoes. Now, he's fit and feeling better than ever.

Growing up, Robert was a proud member of the clean-plate club. Polishing off a large meal earned him praise from his parents, whom he so much wanted to please.

It also earned him a lot of extra weight. By the time he completed his first year of college, he carried 15st 5lb on his 6-foot frame. "I wasn't obese, but I was definitely overweight and seriously out of shape," says 36-year-old Robert.

A year later, Robert dropped out of college for financial reasons. He also moved out of his parents' home. For Robert, these changes signalled a fresh start – an opportunity to redirect his life. Inspired, he set his sights on slimming down.

But not everyone shared Robert's confidence that he could lose weight. His then-girlfriend teased that he was so out of shape that he couldn't run even a mile. "I had to prove to her and to myself that I could do it," he says.

So every evening, Robert went to a local track to run. "I chose running because I wanted an activity that was physically challenging," he explains. "I'd run as long as I could, then walk for a bit, then run again."

As the weeks passed, he could feel himself going further and faster. He was hooked.

In running, Robert found the emotional release that he had once derived from food. It cleared his head of stress and gave him time alone to think through problems and come up with positive ways to solve them. As he continued running and developed healthier eating habits, his weight dropped. He was down to 12st 2lb within 6 months.

Even though he has maintained his weight for 16 years, Robert refuses to take his trim physique for granted. "I must work constantly to balance food and stress with exercise and relaxation, but my efforts have paid off," he says.

And he remains an avid runner – only now he's doing marathons. He has competed in more than 50 races.

WINNING ACTION ➤ ➤ ➤

When you're under stress, run or walk away from the problem.
Physical activity triggers the release of feel-good brain chemicals
called endorphins, giving you a sense of well-being that counteracts
the effects of stress and quashes the urge to overeat. Besides running
when you're under pressure, take a break with walking, swimming,
cycling – anything that gets your body moving.

FEEL GOOD
ABOUT YOU

HER "DREAM BOOK"
WISHES CAME TRUE

For years, Sonia Turner went to bed wanting to lose weight and woke up wanting to lose weight.

"Desire wasn't the problem. What I lacked was the belief that I really could lose weight," recalls Sonia, a 43-year-old estate agent. "I decided that before I could change my body, I had to change my way of thinking."

In January 1997, when she weighed 20st 5lb, Sonia started a scrapbook called *My Dream Book*. In it, she pasted images of people exercising, news stories of people overcoming adversity and, most significant, a photograph from her husband's company newsletter showing a trim-looking, smiling couple at a Christmas party.

Sonia and her husband hadn't gone to that party. "I wanted to stay at home because I was embarrassed," she says. "I cut out that picture and said, 'Next year, we're going.'"

For several weeks, Sonia listened to motivational tapes and pored over the classic book *The Power of Positive Thinking*. Finally, she felt ready to address eating and exercise.

Sonia wanted a plan for life, not just a diet. She evaluated her eating habits and started making more sensible food choices. She took up walking and as the pounds came off, she graduated to jogging. She also signed up for TOPS (Take Off Pounds Sensibly), which provides group support to its members.

By the time the holidays rolled around, Sonia had lost

135 pounds. She and her husband went to the company Christmas party and danced the night away.

Now, her sights are set even higher: she wants to run a marathon. "To be able to run is an unbelievable experience," she says. "I just fell in love with it."

Her dream book remains central to her motivation. Only this time, it's packed full of pictures of runners crossing the finish line.

WINNING ACTION ➤ ➤ ➤

Learn how to believe in yourself. Not all of us grow up with a positive sense of self or the belief that we can get what we really want. Sometimes, we have to learn those important lessons from others. Some of my favourite sources of motivation are Anthony Robbins's Awaken the Giant Within, Oprah Winfrey's Make the Connection and Jon Kabat-Zinn's Full Catastrophe Living. And like Sonia, we should go ahead and dream. After all, dreams do come true.

HER "SMALL" SURPRISE WAS TOPS

In 1997, when David Zimmerman arrived home after a year of active duty overseas in the Marines, he got the surprise of his life. His wife, Hope, was there to greet him – 121 pounds lighter.

He didn't recognise her. He'd never seen her so svelte.

"It was a big motivator for me, to try to shock him," Hope says. And shock him she did. "He didn't know who I was at first," recalls 31-year-old Hope. "After he hugged me, he stepped back to look at me and said, 'Oh my gosh, how did you get smaller than me?' That whole day, he kept touching me now and then, saying, 'I just don't understand where it all went!'"

Hope had set out on her secret weight-loss mission after watching her obese grandmother struggle after breaking a rib. "She was so overweight that it took two people to move her out of bed," Hope recalls. "And she was so independent. I could see what it was doing to her pride. I didn't want that to be me one day."

So at 6 foot and 21st 12lb and with her husband far away, Hope joined TOPS – Take Off Pounds Sensibly. Through the sound diet-and-exercise programme, she whittled her way to 13st 3lb in just over 11 months.

Months later, still excited by her weight-loss success, Hope bought herself a sexy velvet dress. Her husband was on the phone to a relative when she walked downstairs to model it. He paused to lavish her with compliments, then described to the caller how fabulous his wife looked. "The reply was, 'She's not as thin as your brother's girlfriend,'" Hope recalls. "I was devastated."

Hurt and angry, she headed to the kitchen for some solace. But she stopped in her tracks, then went outside for a walk instead. Thirty minutes later, she returned home, calm and enlightened. "I let go of those hurtful words by focusing on the kindness that I received from others who supported me," she says.

Eventually, Hope began strength training to shape and tone her body. Now a Zena-esque size 12 and 13st 13lb, she no longer turns to food to heal those emotional blows. If she feels down, she bypasses the kitchen and heads out for a walk.

WINNING ACTION ➤ ➤ ➤

Realise that you have weight-loss friends and foes. When hurtful words hit you, consider the source. Understand that there will always be negative people in your life, but don't accept their perception of you.

SMALL STEPS LEAD TO BIG WIN

Just one change is all that 36-year-old Julie May needed to kick start her weight-loss programme. And she eventually took off 50 stubborn pounds, one change at a time.

Julie, a hospital case manager, had been trapped in a cycle of dieting, depression and weight gain for most of her adult life. Stung by each failed attempt to slim down, she sought solace in food . . . and put on a pound or two more. Inevitably, she launched new diets, starting the cycle all over again. When her weight reached 13st 8lb, she decided that she'd had enough of her destructive eating pattern.

In search of a solution to her weight-loss woes, Julie picked up a copy of Oprah Winfrey's best-seller *Make the Connection*. As she read about Winfrey's struggle to slim down, Julie made a connection of her own. "I had tried and failed on so many diets that I no longer believed that I could lose weight," she says. "I had to prove to myself that I could succeed." She would do that by making one change at a time.

Julie decided to work on her activity level first since she knew that her eating habits would be harder to change. She set a goal of walking for 20 minutes, 4 days a week. As her fitness improved, she found that she could go longer. Within a matter of weeks, when she actually looked forward to her regular walks, she knew that she had succeeded in making exercise a part of her life.

Excited by her progress, Julie felt ready to tackle her eating habits. Her first step was to phase out the sweets, biscuits and desserts that had once been her comfort foods. She didn't tell herself that she couldn't have sweets; instead, when she indulged, she reminded herself that what she was eating could impede her weight-loss efforts. Within a month, she was making conscious decisions to *not* eat the chocolate cake or lemon meringue pie that she had once thought she couldn't pass up.

Julie continued to improve her eating habits, eating more fruits and vegetables, paring her fat intake and portion sizes and drinking more water. She made one change at a time, allowing herself time to adapt before moving on to something new. "I never felt overwhelmed," she says. "And each success made me more and more confident that I could lose weight."

Julie did lose weight – 50 pounds, to be exact. And she has kept off the weight for a year and a half.

As a bonus, her mental attitude and energy are at an all-time high.

WINNING ACTION ➤ ➤ ➤

Make one change and give it a chance. As Julie illustrated so well, one small achievement will lead to the next. In fact, weight-loss experts have observed that it takes about 6 weeks for any lifestyle change to become a habit. So allow yourself the time to adjust. If you slip up by eating a dozen doughnuts in one sitting or skipping your workout for 2 days in a row, don't beat yourself up over it. Just pick up where you left off. Before you know it, your healthy new behaviour will seem like second nature to you.

SHE FOUND THE SUPPORT SHE NEEDED

At 29, Olivia Williamson found out she had high blood pressure. Her doctor told her that unless she did something about it, she could be on drugs for the rest of her life.

Olivia knew what that "something" was. After all, she weighed 17st 2lb. "I had no choice but to slim down. Having high blood pressure really scared me," she says.

It's not that she hadn't tried before. Diet and exercise regimes were no strangers to Olivia. But she could never stick with them on her own. This time, she decided, she'd enlist help.

Luckily for Olivia, her employer, a university, offers a 6-week healthy-weight-management class through the school's medical centre. Once the class is over, students can attend weekly support-group meetings for up to 4 months. Olivia signed on.

For the first 10 weeks, she diligently followed the directions of the class instructor, cutting back on fat, eating less in one sitting and exercising moderately. But she didn't lose a single pound. Was she frustrated? You bet. But the support group kept Olivia going.

"Just being able to tell the group, 'I'm doing it; I'm sticking with it' made me feel better," says Olivia. "It allowed me to settle in to the healthier habits that I was learning." She enjoyed the group so much that when her weight-management course ended, she joined an e-mail diet-support network she found through the university.

Within a year, Olivia lost 45 pounds and her blood pressure returned to a healthy level. As a bonus, she had more energy than ever before, which encouraged her to stay active in her daily life. "When I went on a sight-seeing trip around Europe in 1999, I was able to climb all 340 steps to the top of Notre Dame Cathedral," she says. "I wouldn't have been able to do that before!"

WINNING ACTION ➤➤➤

Develop a network of weight-loss friends. In a support group, you meet people who are facing the exact same challenges as you. It's a perfect forum for exchanging advice on what works and what doesn't, for unloading your frustrations and for celebrating your victories. To locate a support group near you, start by checking with local libraries, hospitals and churches. Or check whether your employer keeps a list of local resources.

LOVE GAVE HER A LIFT

When Debbie Watson didn't feel good about her life, she turned to food for a quick fix. Bingeing lessened her isolation and pain, but at the expense of her waistline. Only when she learned to love herself and accept love from others did she succeed in slimming down.

Debbie traces her struggle with bingeing to her father's death when she was only 16. "I felt empty and I tried to fill that emptiness with food," she explains. When she went away to college 2 years later, her sadness and loneliness only got worse. "I gained about 25 pounds in my first couple of years away from home," she says.

She managed to take off most of the extra weight while still in college, primarily by watching what she ate. As she got slimmer, her self-esteem improved. But it didn't last.

By the time she reached her late twenties, Debbie was in the throes of another personal crisis. "Basically, I didn't know what I wanted to do with my life and I turned to food for comfort," she says. "I'd eat until I physically hurt, then I'd lie on the sofa until the pain went away."

Looking back, Debbie attributes her overeating to her desire for control. "I felt powerless in so many areas of my life," she explains. "But I had power over food. I could do with it whatever I wanted."

The repeated binges drove Debbie's weight upwards. By 30, she reached 12st 12lb. "I felt awful about myself and that only made me eat more," she recalls.

Debbie knew that she couldn't continue her erratic eating habits without seriously undermining her health. Determined to get to the bottom of her binges, she decided to join Overeaters Anonymous (OA). There, she began to uncover why she used food to fill voids in her life. She learned better ways of coping with her sadness and loneliness, such as calling a friend on the phone. Most important, she recognised her own strengths and attributes, gradually accepting her value as a person.

It was a painful process, but other members of the OA group gave Debbie support and understanding. "I'll always be grateful to them for standing by me," she says. "They not only helped me overcome my loneliness but also taught me how to deal with food."

What's more, Debbie's positive interactions with other OA members gave her the courage to cultivate friendships outside the group, with her neighbours and colleagues. "As I allowed people into my life, I felt less lonely and much happier," she says. "I no longer needed food as an emotional crutch."

With the OA group's guidance and encouragement, Debbie began to transform her eating habits. As Debbie's eating habits and self-image improved, her bingeing subsided. She was able to drop 30 pounds in about 8 months. Fifteen years later, she's still holding steady at a healthy 10st 10lb.

Debbie believes that self-acceptance gave her the incentive to adopt a healthier lifestyle. "A lot of overweight people feel bad about themselves and they won't let themselves love who they are," she explains. "But once you love yourself, you can give love to others and receive love in return. That gives you a sense of fulfilment that you won't ever get from overeating."

WINNING ACTION ➤ ➤ ➤

Accept and appreciate yourself just as you are. When you're not feeling good about yourself or some aspect of your life, you may turn to food to lift your spirits. It works, but it's only a temporary fix that will probably leave you feeling worse in the long run. So don't beat yourself up by bingeing. Instead, cultivate a sense of self-acceptance and self-respect that can get you through the tough times. Try making a list of all that's good about you and your life, then read it over and over again as needed for a major ego boost.

LEAN AND LOVING IT

When Carol Haas was 17 years old, she began forcing herself to vomit after meals in a desperate and dangerous attempt to slim down. At 5 foot 8 inches and 11st 6lb, the high-school athlete was hardly obese. But her self-image had taken such a beating as a result of a lifetime of painful personal problems that she became fixated on her weight.

So began a 20-year struggle with eating disorders that dragged Carol through episodes of anorexia, bingeing and purging, excessive dieting and compulsive exercising. "I felt awful about myself and what I was doing," says the 57 year old. "But I couldn't stop myself. I was out of control. I was determined to not be fat, regardless of the price I paid."

It took the demise of a troubled first marriage and the understanding and concern of the man who would become her second husband, to finally free Carol from the eating disorders that had plagued her for so long. With encouragement from her new partner, she sought counselling to help her deal with the issues that had skewed her self-image and her attitude towards food and eating.

Through her counselling sessions, Carol came to understand the reasons for her eating disorder. She learned that she had to take control of her eating habits rather than let them control her. She gradually adapted to eating three healthy meals a day and exercising regularly – not compulsively.

"During my recovery, one of the most important things I did was allow myself foods that I had always considered off-limits," Carol says. "That empowered me because I realised I could choose what to eat and what not to eat.

"There's dignity in choice," she adds. "It explodes self-imposed boundaries. It puts you in charge. It gives you freedom and power over food. For someone with an eating disorder, that's a life-altering and often life-saving revelation."

It certainly had a profound impact on Carol. As she made peace with food, her self-image improved. She began to heal, physically and emotionally. And, to her pleasant surprise, she lost 20 pounds over the course of 2 years.

A few years later, Carol enrolled in college to earn certification as an eating disorders counsellor. "I was so grateful for my own recovery that I wanted to help others," she explains.

"My life changed dramatically when I finally stopped my power struggle with food," Carol says. "I was able to focus on being healthy instead of on what I was or wasn't eating. That has made all the difference."

WINNING ACTION ➤ ➤ ➤

Get to the root of the problem. Eating disorders often arise from underlying personal issues that chip away at a person's self-image. They're the sorts of issues that advice about eating right and exercising just won't resolve. If you suspect that you have an eating disorder, get help. Your local hospital may be able to refer you to qualified therapists and support groups in your area.

NOTHING COMES BETWEEN HER AND HER WORKOUTS

Everyone in Regina Owens's life understands that nothing interferes with her workouts. After all, it was this kind of passion and devotion that enabled her to lose 65 pounds and reduce her dress size from a 24 to a 12.

Each day, Regina rises at 4:30 a.m. for a 5-mile walk. In the evening, after work, she packs herself and her kids in the car and drives 30 miles to a gym. While she lifts weights for an hour, her kids do their homework.

"Yes, I'm obsessive. But at least the whole exercise thing is a healthy obsession for me. That hasn't always been so," says Regina, a 46-year-old housing director.

Indeed, before Regina latched on to exercise, she was eating too much and abusing sleeping pills – her ways of coping with the emotional strain of a difficult marriage.

Turning her life around required that she pursue health as obsessively as she once had those destructive behaviours. "I needed to do something positive and I needed to do it whole-heartedly," she says.

She began by taking long walks around a lake near her home. During those walks, she thought about her problems and her desire to change. Within a few months, she was averaging between 8 and 10 miles a day. She began eating better, too, by reducing her fat intake, restricting sweets and learning to control her compulsive snacking. She took up weightlifting and studied to become a certified trainer, which she now does as a sideline.

"To succeed, I knew I had to go at it full force," she says. "Later, my motivation came from seeing my body go through this incredible transformation. I got leaner and fitter.

"Once that started happening, my workouts became something I needed to do," she says. "Now, if I don't get my workout in, I don't feel like my day is complete."

WINNING ACTION ➤➤➤

Work with your personality, not against it. Concentrate on turning negative obsessions and behaviours into healthy passions and choices. Be obsessive, but in a positive way, if that suits your personality. If you're more laid-back, focus on making small changes. Find the style that works for you.

SETBACKS DIDN'T GET IN HER WAY

In a roundabout way, Sandra Wadsworth credits her dry cleaner with motivating her to lose weight.

"In 1993, I finally accepted that my dry cleaner wasn't shrinking my clothes," laughs the 41 year old. "And I admitted to myself that my zips weren't breaking because my clothes were poorly made."

Sandy knew that, at 10st 10lb, she was heavier than she had ever been, because her eating habits were out of control. But every time she tried to lose weight, she quit as soon as she made even the most minor mistake, like choosing a "bad" food or eating too much. Embarrassed by her inability to stick with a weight-loss programme, she refused to discuss her problem with her family or closest friends.

Eventually, Sandy sought help from Weight Watchers, thinking that a structured approach to weight loss might be what she needed. Through the programme, she learned how emotional upsets such as boredom and stress drove her to binge on junk food and fast food. "I also became aware of my habit of 'unconscious eating' – munching on a handful of M&M's at work and not remembering whose sweet jar I had raided," she says.

Even more important to Sandy was the rebirth of her self-esteem. "Weight Watchers helped me see that I wasn't a bad person because I was overweight," she says. "I just needed to learn healthy eating habits."

After 5 months in the programme, Sandy lost 20 pounds. She has stayed at her goal weight of 9st 4lb for more than 5 years.

Sandy admits that she has had her share of slip-ups. The difference is that she no longer views every setback as a failure. "Everyone makes mistakes," she says. "The key to weight-loss success is turning each mistake into a learning experience."

WINNING ACTION ➤➤➤

Challenge all-or-nothing thinking. *So you ate a half-pound of your favourite chocolates. That doesn't mean that you failed, that you're a bad person or that your diet is over. Acknowledge the blip and just pick up where you left off. Even the most successful "losers" slip up. That's called being human. The trick is to learn from the situation and keep trying. Remember, every day really is a new day.*

WEIGHT LOSS WAS JUST A HAIRCUT AWAY

Over the course of 14 years, Kelly Feick lost and regained between 80 and 140 pounds five times. Then, a haircut changed her life.

Kelly was the kind of girl who got a lot of compliments on her hair. Blond and thick, flowing to her waist, it hadn't been cut in 14 years. It seemed to be the only thing that people noticed about her. And at 22st 7lb, the young nurse was glad. She liked to believe that her hair hid her body.

But by the time she turned 28, Kelly was a mess, physically and emotionally. She couldn't look into the mirror without crying. Every joint in her body ached. Bitterness began to show in her features. She realised that she needed to renew her weight-loss efforts. More important, she needed the results to stick. She vowed to change her life, not just her weight.

To do this, Kelly decided to take a risk so drastic that it would prove her commitment to her efforts. "I knew that if I could handle getting my hair cut off, I could get through anything," she says. And cut off her hair she did, all the way to the middle of her neck.

The change sparked a sense of purpose and commitment in Kelly. She began making better food choices, cooking healthier and walking every day. In just 1 year, she lost 185 pounds.

These days, Kelly is letting her hair grow back a little. But those pounds have stayed away.

WINNING ACTION ➤ ➤ ➤

Throw away your security blanket. As Kelly discovered, making a major non-weight-related change can serve as a stepping stone to permanent weight loss. Think of something daring that you've always wanted to try – even something as radical as bungee jumping or skydiving. Meeting a challenge builds your self-confidence and makes you feel empowered: "If I can do that, I can do anything!"

REFLECTING ON WEIGHT-LOSS SUCCESS

When Adrienne Sussman's sister-in-law lost weight, it was the proverbial straw that broke the camel's back. "I had always been thinner and fitter than she was," explains 52-year-old Adrienne. "Now, she looked better than me."

Envious of her sister-in-law's success, Adrienne was determined to get back her former shapely figure. A svelte 17st 5lb for most of her life, she began to gain weight after giving birth to her son in 1984. Once he started nursery school at 2, Adrienne turned to food to make her feel better. "I missed my son so much and felt so guilty for sending him to school that I started eating just to calm my nerves," she recalls. "I went to the bakery every day to buy a pastry for myself, one for my husband and one for my son. Then, I'd eat all three."

Within a year and a half, Adrienne's weight rose to 9st 13lb. "At that point, my self-esteem had hit rock bottom," she explains. "I looked in the mirror and I really didn't like what I saw." Ironically, that mirror would later become a critical component of Adrienne's weight-loss programme.

Determined to get rid of her excess baggage, Adrienne signed up for Weight Watchers. "My sister-in-law had joined and I figured that if she could do it, I could do it," she explains. But it wasn't easy at first. "I didn't want to go to the weekly meetings, because I felt really self-conscious," she says. "So I wrote 'doctor's appointment' on my calendar to fool myself into attending." Eventually, she started looking forward to the meetings, where she learned to use a combination of portion control, exercise and behaviour modification to slim down.

To monitor her progress, every couple of weeks she'd stand in front of the mirror completely naked and do a head-to-toe body check. Over the next few months, she saw her body changing. That's what kept her motivated. "I stopped looking in the mirror and telling myself that I was destined to be overweight forever," she says. "I accepted that whatever was broken, I had the power to fix."

With this new, positive attitude, Adrienne was able to shed 30 pounds. She has maintained her weight at a healthy 7st 11lb for 8 years.

These days, Adrienne serves as a programme leader for Weight Watchers. She constantly reminds people in her group to stop obsessing about the number on the scales. "The most important questions you should ask yourself are, 'Are you happy with what you look like? Do you like the way you perceive yourself? And do you like the way you carry yourself?'" she says. "It's what you think when you look in the mirror – not the number on the scales – that matters."

WINNING ACTION ➤ ➤ ➤

Let your mirror be your friend. Self-acceptance – even when you're naked – is an important first step of any weight-loss programme. Once you feel comfortable with yourself, you'll have the confidence and patience to achieve lasting weight-loss success. Try the same strategy that worked for Adrienne: every 2 weeks or so, take off your clothes and stand in front of a mirror completely nude. At first, you may not like what you see. But find one part that you do like, even if it's your elbows! Over time, as your body changes, you'll find more to like and you'll continue your weight-loss efforts.

SHE USED HER MIND TO SLIM HER BODY

After years of dieting, Leigh Anne Congdon finally took off – and kept off – 30 pounds. She did it, she says, by learning how to think like a thin person.

As a teenager, Leigh Anne was unhappy with her body. She was only a few pounds overweight, but she saw herself as chunky and unattractive. She'd go on self-styled diets of less than 1,000 calories a day for a couple of weeks at a time and she would lose a few pounds. But once she had returned to her normal eating habits, the weight would always come back.

This cycle of gaining, losing and regaining continued through school and college. Then, Leigh Anne made a decision that would turn her eating habits upside down. "When I graduated, I moved to a new city with a group of friends," she explains. "I thought that I could find a job there and I was excited about living in another part of the country. I needed the change."

Away from home and living with her friends, Leigh Anne

decided to enjoy herself. That meant not worrying all the time about what she was eating. She joined her friends in a steady diet of pizza, burgers, barbecued ribs and other foods of which she had deprived herself for so long. Within a year, her weight climbed from 10 stone to 11st 6lb – too heavy for her 5-foot-5-inch frame.

Once again, Leigh Anne decided that it was time for a fresh start. "It wasn't only my weight," she says. "It was the part-time jobs, the small flats. I needed some direction in my life."

She headed back home and enrolled on a post-graduate course. And she committed to slimming down healthily and permanently.

Remembering how dieting had failed her in the past, but not wanting to monitor every bite of food that she put in her mouth, Leigh Anne decided to change her mindset. "I had noticed that my friends who were thin didn't constantly dwell on what they were eating," she explains. "They ate when they were hungry and said, 'No, thanks' when they weren't. I followed their example and tried to stop obsessing about food. I resolved to think like a thin person."

Leigh Anne played the part of a thin person on a daily basis. "When I'd get up in the morning, I'd remind myself to think like a thin person," she says. "I'd eat a little bit of something and then tell myself that I was full, because that's what a thin person would do." She ate more healthily, too, replacing those burgers and ribs with vegetarian meals and salads.

Leigh Anne also increased her activity level, believing that a thin person would be active. She took up hiking and she rode her bike instead of driving her car.

With her new "thin" attitude, Leigh Anne was able to take off 30 pounds in about 9 months. Now aged 42, she has maintained her weight at a healthy 9st 4lb ever since.

WINNING ACTION ➤ ➤ ➤

Think – then act – like a thin person. *By thinking of yourself as a thin, active, healthy person, you empower yourself to do what's necessary to become that person. Do it right now: close your eyes and create a mental image of yourself as you want to be. Pay attention to details. Where are you? How do you look? What are you wearing? How do you feel? Study the image for about 10 minutes, then open your eyes. Invoke that image as often as you like throughout the day. It can be a powerful motivator.*

SHE BROKE A 50-YEAR BINGE CYCLE

Joyce Perata distinctly remembers her first eating binge. An ice cream van was passing through her neighbourhood and she ran out to buy a supply of her favourite treat: choc ices. She ran back home, sat on the kitchen floor and devoured the 3 or 4 ices one after another.

At the time, she was all of 9 years old.

Joyce had been living with her grandmother until that summer, when she moved in with her parents. "Because both of them worked during the day, I found myself home alone, missing my grandmother," she recalls. "Eating was my way of comforting myself.

"I learned at an early age to use food to deal with my emotions, whether I was feeling lonely, anxious or sad," says the 56 year old. "Eating was an antidote to my negative feelings and my lack of self-worth. It numbed me."

It also precipitated Joyce's nearly half-century struggle with her weight, which careered between a high of 12st 2lb and a low of 7 stone on her 5-foot-2-inch frame. In college, Joyce smoked to stay thin. In her thirties, she sucked down diet pills. In her forties, she began eating healthily, walking and doing aerobics. But when her marriage fell apart, she once again turned to food for comfort.

Finally, at 54, Joyce had had enough. "I had been getting help from a psychiatrist in working through my occasional bouts of bulimia and anorexia," she says. "My psychiatrist suggested that I join Honesty, Openness and Willingness, an offshoot organisation of Overeaters Anonymous." The programme taught Joyce how to control her bingeing and gave her tools to deal with the emotions that drove her to food in the first place. Through the organisation, Joyce says, she discovered an inner clarity and peace that she had never before experienced. For the first time in her life, she felt good about herself, without the aid of food. "I learned to accept my body as it is without trying to be skinny," she says. "I could look in the mirror and feel okay about myself."

Empowered, Joyce consulted a nutritionist to learn how to eat better. She also resumed her exercise programme. As a result of her healthier lifestyle, she has lost 8 stone.

For Joyce, even more valuable than her weight loss is her newfound self-confidence and self-esteem. "Now, I recognise my feelings," she says, "and I feel joy and freedom."

WINNING ACTION ➤ ➤ ➤

Feed emotional hunger without food. Like Joyce, you may have a strong emotional attachment to food and bingeing that's so complex that you need professional guidance to work through it. Don't be embarrassed and don't let feelings of shame or pride ("I should be able to beat this alone") keep you from seeking help. That's what the pros are there for – to help people like you and me unravel the years of habit that have made food our emotional salve for hurt and low self-worth. Find a counsellor whom you trust and start feeling better today. If you need incentive to take that first step, think about how it helped Joyce.

HUMILIATION TURNS TO 65 POUNDS OF DETERMINATION

Lori LaRizzio found the willpower to forgo fast food once her weight-loss success became an issue of pride, money and her best friend's wedding.

At the age of 30, Lori seemed to have everything: the love of her husband, two great kids, a wonderful career in nursing. But at 5 foot 5 inches and 14st 9lb, she hated her body – and shopping for clothes. To avoid feeling humiliated, she looked at handbags and earrings while her friends tried on miniskirts and bikinis.

But humiliation was exactly what Lori felt when she was fitted for a bridesmaid's dress for her best friend's wedding. The seamstress shouted out Lori's 44-37-45 measurements for all to hear. Then she said brassily, "You'll need to pay more. You're too big for regular sizes."

Sobbing, Lori headed straight for McDonald's to indulge in chips and a sundae, her favourite comfort foods. But by the time she got there, she had changed her mind. She bought a diet Coke and drove home, where she immediately called the seamstress and ordered a smaller size. The woman argued. Lori insisted.

Five months and lots of low-fat meals, walks and bicycle rides later, Lori got her sweet revenge. The seamstress had to take in Lori's size-16 gown.

Since her friend's wedding, Lori's efforts to slim down have continued to pay off. She's down to 10 stone, a weight that she has maintained for more than 3 years.

"Despite her rudeness, I actually have to thank that seamstress," Lori says. "She catapulted me to a new, healthier way of living."

TOWN WATCHED AS SHE LOST POUNDS

When Debbie Owen decided to lose weight, she invited the readers of the newspaper in her hometown – all 500,000 of them – to cheer her on.

Even with her supporters, Debbie understood that there was only one way she would slim down successfully: she had to do it for herself. And she did, losing 91 pounds in 18 months.

Debbie, a 42-year-old marketing manager, had struggled with her weight since secondary school. "I went on every kind of diet known to womankind," she says. When she reached 20st 6lb, she despaired that she'd never achieve a healthy weight.

When her husband suggested they start exercising to an aerobics video every night, she reluctantly decided to join him. She admits that her heart wasn't in it – until she noticed that her clothes were looser after just 3 weeks of working out. Inspired, she decided to give weight loss one more try.

Ever the marketing professional, Debbie wondered whether her story had any publicity potential for the newspaper that employed her. So she proposed that a reporter chronicle her quest.

Once a month, the newspaper ran an article on her progress. It also set up a special voice-mail number so that readers could leave messages for Debbie. "I heard from all kinds of people – husbands who wanted their wives to lose weight, teenagers, even people from outside the paper's readership area," she says. They offered their encouragement and asked for her suggestions on weight loss.

While grateful for the support of her husband and the strangers who followed her story in the newspaper, Debbie kept reminding herself that she was slimming down for her sake and no one else's. "If you lose weight for another person, you start to look for feedback from that person," she explains. "If you do it because you want to please your husband but he doesn't seem to notice, you don't get the reward you expected. But if you do it for yourself, the reward comes from within you. That's when you start to succeed."

With 91 pounds gone, Debbie is still working towards her goal weight of 12st 7lb. She feels so good about herself that she's confident of her ability to go all the way.

WINNING ACTION ➤ ➤ ➤

Create a support group, but listen to yourself. Enlist the support of family members, friends and even neighbours and colleagues by telling them about your weight-loss goals. But don't let their support – or lack thereof – be your only guide. Be clear on why you want to lose the weight. In life, you need to please yourself.

A LITTLE COACHING MADE HER A WEIGHT-LOSS WINNER

Jeanann Pock isn't what you'd call a morning person. But with a little help from legendary American football coach Vince Lombardi, she found a way to resist the snooze alarm. She ended up losing 85 pounds as a result.

In 1992, Jeanann was a 22-year-old graduate about to embark on a career in university public affairs. At 5 foot 2 inches and 14st 4lb – she gained about 20 pounds in each of her last 3 years of college – she wondered whether she would be able to meet the demands of her new job. "Being overweight made everyday activities so much more tiring than they used to be," she explains. "I made up my mind to slim down."

Armed with information from the university library, Jeanann began trimming the fat from her diet and walking on a daily basis. She planned her walks for first thing in the morning so she'd be certain to fit them into her schedule. The trouble was that she had a hard time getting up early. At 4:45 a.m., all she wanted to do was snooze.

At about that time, Jeanann happened to be reading *What It Takes to Be Number One*, a book by Vince Lombardi. She was struck by one particular passage, in which Lombardi wrote, "Winning is not a sometime thing; it's an all-the-time thing."

His words provided the motivation that Jeanann needed. "I understood that to succeed at weight loss, I had to win every little battle along the way – including my morning skirmishes with my alarm clock," she says. "I had to think like a winner to be a winner."

From that point on, Jeanann had a new morning ritual. Rather than hiding her head under her pillow to block out her alarm clock's ring, she repeated to herself Lombardi's words. And then she asked herself, "Do I really want to be fat?" That got her out of bed and into her running shoes.

It also kept her weight-loss programme on track. "After all, a winner doesn't give up when she's halfway to the finish line," Jeanann says. Within a year, she got rid of all 85 unwanted pounds. She has maintained her weight at a healthy 8st 3lb ever since.

SHE'S SAVOURING WEIGHT-LOSS SUCCESS

Jill Scoggins was on her way to weight-loss success. Then, a new job, a new home and a family wedding nearly derailed her efforts. But she managed to get back on track, eventually losing 37 stubborn pounds.

Her secret? She concentrated on her accomplishments rather than dwelling on her defeats.

Jill, 41, says that she never worried much about her weight, not even as her dress size got bigger. "I suppose that I was in denial," she explains. "It was a very gradual gain, so it was easy for me to ignore." But when her size-16 clothes – what she calls her fat clothes – started feeling tight, she decided that she had to slim down. And she knew exactly what to do: eat better, drink lots of water and, for the first time in her life, exercise.

Jill launched her weight-loss programme in September 1998. She concentrated on making healthier food choices while phasing out late-night snacking. She also joined a gym and consulted a personal trainer, who helped her develop an exercise programme that included aerobic workouts and strength training.

Jill's plan worked perfectly. Within 1 month, she lost 8 pounds. "That convinced me that I could lose even more," she says. "So I kept at it and the more I lost, the more I wanted to stick with it."

She managed to stick with it for 4 months, taking off another 27 pounds. Then, her life turned upside down. Both she and her husband landed new jobs further from home. When they weren't commuting, they were house hunting. In what little spare time she had left, Jill was helping her stepdaughter plan her wedding.

With her schedule crammed, Jill's weight-loss programme stalled. "I didn't have time to go to the gym or even to pack my lunch," she says. "I found myself in fast-food restaurants more often than I care to admit."

Jill could feel herself getting discouraged. "I was still losing weight, but at a much slower rate," she explains. But then, she remembered how faithfully she had followed her programme and how easily the pounds had been coming off. "I told myself, 'You've proven that you can lose weight. Just do what you have to do,'" she says.

Her personal pep talk paid off. Within a year of starting her weight-loss programme, Jill dropped 37 pounds and four dress sizes. She has maintained her weight at 8st 8lb ever since. She and her husband eventually found a new home and her stepdaughter's wedding went off without a hitch. "Many of the guests commented on my weight loss," she says. "That made me feel great!"

WINNING ACTION ➤ ➤ ➤

Remember your victories. Revel in your successes, no matter how small they may seem. Today, you may be only 1 pound lighter. In 6 months, that 1 pound could be 50! Acknowledge every step that you make towards weight-loss success. Knowing that you can slim down will keep you motivated when your determination starts to wane.

A TAPE RECORDER TOOK
HER FROM BOTTOM TO TOP

Beth Linden remembers meeting her little daughter's new friend as if it were yesterday. "She looked at my daughter and said, 'I didn't know your mummy was fat,'" the 39 year old recalls.

It was the worst – and, as it turned out, the best – moment of her life.

Devastated by the remark, Beth – then aged 30 and 17st 2lb – took out a tape recorder and started talking about how she felt. She stated the date and her height and weight. Then she let loose. Her voice quivering, she described the incident with her daughter's friend. How she hated putting her daughter in such an awkward situation. How lonely and empty she felt. What it meant and felt like to be so heavy. How the laces hung on the sides of her shoes because she was too fat to bend down to tie them. How embarrassed she was to buy clothes. She said she hated the way she looked. She hated herself.

Calmed by the emotional release, Beth dried her eyes and, with more determination than ever, decided to do something about her weight. She studied all the official nutritional guidelines to learn how to eat more healthily. She cut back on fatty foods and ate lots of fresh fruits and vegetables when she felt hungry. And she walked for 30 minutes every day – outside when she could, inside on her treadmill when the weather was bad. It took 2 years, but she lost 100 pounds.

Four years later, she needed the tape again. "I had gained 15 pounds and my eating habits were terrible," she says. "When I played the tape, I could hear the rain outside and the desperation in my voice. I was only 34 years old and I didn't want to go back." It immediately turned her around.

Now Beth plays the same tape every year around October 1 to gear herself up for the Christmas holidays. This autumn ritual and the stinging remembrance of a little girl's remark have helped to kept her weight under 10st 10lb for more than 5 years.

WINNING ACTION ➤ ➤ ➤

Use your low point for inspiration. In a journal, on a tape recorder or just on a piece of paper, make a record of exactly why you want to lose weight at that low moment. Describe in detail how you feel and what you want to change. Read it over or listen to it when you're tempted to fall off the weight-loss wagon. And, like Beth, hang on to it for the future, as a reminder of how far you've come. (I still have a few fat drawings that I made of myself more than 10 years ago!)

SHE DISCOVERED HER HIPS AT THE AGE OF 33

In 1987, Fay Hodge stepped onto the scales at a Weight Watchers meeting. It was the first step of a journey in which she would lose 111 pounds and find a tremendous power within herself: the power to choose.

Fay had struggled with her weight since childhood, when she was taught to eat everything on her plate. "My grandmother used to say that what I didn't finish at dinner, she'd scramble the next morning," she recalls. "She was teasing, but I got the message. My family worked hard to put food on the table. My job was to eat it."

Unfortunately, the combination of eating too much and exercising too little quickly took its toll. At 7, Fay was put on her first diet by her doctor. It didn't work. Neither did the diets that followed. She just kept gaining. At 33, she weighed 19 stone – "I was uncomfortable in my own skin and getting ready to develop another set of stretch marks," she says.

At the time, a friend of Fay's was going to Weight Watchers and she urged Fay to join, too. It was through the organisation's weekly meetings that Fay came to a profound realisation: her weight and her health are the culmination of countless choices that she makes every day.

"I can choose to eat the right foods in the right portions and be successful or I can choose to eat foods and portions that will cause weight gain," she explains. "The decision is mine. I'm in control."

With a newfound sense of empowerment, Fay embraced the Weight Watchers principles, eating a wider variety of nutritious foods, monitoring her portion control and drinking lots of water. She also increased her level of physical activity by walking briskly three or four times a week. And sure enough, the weight came off.

"There is nothing more exciting than discovering a hip bone. I felt like Columbus!" she says. "I was absolutely intrigued that there was a body underneath all of those layers."

In just 1 year, Fay took off 111 pounds. And she has kept off the weight for 11 years. Today, at 45, she's a statuesque 5 foot 11 inches and a size 14.

She was so inspired by her own success that she became a Weight Watchers leader, helping others take the first steps of their own weight-loss journeys.

WINNING ACTION ➤ ➤ ➤

It's never too late to lose. When weight gain starts so early in life, it's all that much harder to realise that there is a thin person in there, just begging to come out. Overweight needn't be anyone's destiny. Determination and the realisation that you will succeed is the first step. When you start to doubt, just think of Fay.

STIMULATE YOUR DETERMINATION

SHE PUT FITNESS FIRST AND LOST 155 POUNDS

With a family, a home and a part-time job, Sandie Howe doesn't have a lot of free time. But no matter how busy she is, 34-year-old Sandie sets aside 30 minutes a day, just for herself, to exercise. Her no-excuses attitude towards fitness helped her lose 155 pounds and 10 dress sizes.

Sandie never had a weight problem when she was younger. But once she and her husband decided to start a family, she gained between 35 and 40 pounds with each of her four babies. By 32, she weighed 21st 6lb.

"My mum took a photo of me that Christmas, in 1997," Sandie recalls. "When I saw it, I was so ashamed that I wanted to cry. I made up my mind right then and there to lose weight."

The trouble was that she didn't even know where to start. "In the past, I had made some half-hearted attempts to lose weight, but without much success," she says. "I really didn't know what to do."

She knew from experience that dieting didn't work. So this time, she decided to combine a sensible eating plan with regular exercise. She began counting calories and grams of fat and exercising for 30 minutes at least three times a week. "I really struggled at first," she recalls. "Whether I was walking outside or doing aerobics to a video, I was pretty winded by the time I was done."

As the pounds came off, though, she felt stronger and better. She noticed that her feet and knees, which had bothered her when she was at her heaviest, no longer hurt.

Over time, Sandie expanded her exercise programme so that she was working out for at least 30 minutes every day.

She continued to monitor her calorie and fat intake, too. Within 2 years, she lost 155 pounds. She's now a fit and trim 10st 5lb.

"When it comes to exercising, the biggest excuse is not having time. I know – I used to tell myself that, too," Sandie says. "I learned that I can make time, if I really want to. Some days, I get up a half-hour early, so I can squeeze in my workout before things get hectic. Other days, I exercise while my children are napping or playing at friends' homes. If all else fails, my husband is great about watching the kids so I can go walking for 30 minutes.

"Somehow I always find the time I need," Sandie adds. "You can, too."

WINNING ACTION ➤ ➤ ➤

Make yourself a top priority. No matter how busy a family life you have, follow Sandie's example and demand a half-hour a day for yourself. If your family objects, explain to them how important it is to you and that they'll benefit, too – by having a happier, healthier wife and mother. Out of 24 hours in a day, you deserve 30 minutes!

WEIGHT LOSS WAS A BONUS OF HER CHOLESTEROL CURE

Pam Cook started exercising to beat a family history of heart disease and diabetes. As a bonus, she lost 35 pounds – and she has never looked better or felt better in her life.

But that wasn't the case just 2 years ago, when Pam carried 10st 5lb on her 5-foot frame. She found out that her cholesterol was well above the recommended maximum level.

Worse, her triglycerides – a type of blood fat implicated in heart disease – were much higher than they should have been.

Pam's doctor warned her that if she didn't boost her activity level, she could expect to follow in the footsteps of many of her family members. When Pam confided that she hated to exercise, her doctor suggested that she start walking.

"The first day, I started off slow and didn't go very far," she recalls. "But every day, I went a little bit faster and a little bit further." Soon, she was taking brisk walks every morning and evening. Now, she walks 4 to 6 miles every day around her hometown.

Pam also made some changes in her eating habits, too. "I had talked to my sister-in-law about my cholesterol problem and soon after, she surprised me with a copy of *The Fat-Free Living Super Cookbook* by Jyl Steinback," Pam says. "I used that book as a guide to eliminating all the fat from my meals. The dessert recipes are especially wonderful."

The results have been amazing. Pam's cholesterol level has fallen to acceptable levels and her triglycerides have dropped below the recommended maximum. "My doctor was thrilled," Pam, now 47, says. But that isn't the only thing that's pleased Pam. She's now 35 pounds lighter, thanks to her walking workouts.

WINNING ACTION ➤ ➤ ➤

Do it for your health's sake. Maybe slimming down for appearance's sake isn't enough of a motivator for you. So do it for your health instead. Research has shown that for someone who is overweight, even a modest amount of weight loss – in the order of 10 to 14 pounds – can lower the risk of heart disease and certain cancers, protect against back and joint pain, boost energy and improve sleep.

SHE'S WEARING HER LITTLE BLACK DRESS AGAIN

A little black dress hung from Dinah Burnette's wardrobe door, reminding her of the past and showing her what the future might hold. But at 17st 7lb, she couldn't even pull the dress over her hips.

Being overweight was a new experience for Dinah. When she was a teenager, she stayed trim despite hearty meat-and-potato meals and midnight pizza sessions. And as a young woman, her figure always snapped back after the birth of each of her four children.

But when Dinah was in her late twenties, she added 100 pounds to her frame in just 2 years. During that time, she had started taking a prescription medication that sometimes causes weight gain. But she also suspected that her metabolism had just slowed down.

Even though the clothes in her wardrobe grew bigger and bigger, Dinah didn't acknowledge just how much weight she'd accumulated until she saw photographs of her 1996 nursing-school graduation. "I was in this fantasy world that there were several girls in my class bigger than me," she says. "When that class picture came, I was the biggest. I just remember being so embarrassed."

So she began a self-styled regime of healthy meals, a gallon of water a day and lots of exercise. "When I started, I couldn't even walk a half-mile," she says. "But in 6 months, I worked my way up to 3 miles every day." For motivation, Dinah hung her expensive black dress, the only piece of small-size clothing she'd kept, on her wardrobe door. The last time she had worn it was to a wedding in early 1989.

"I would try it on every 4 weeks and see how close the buttons were getting. Gradually, I could get it on, but the buttons were 4 feet apart," she laughs. One year later and 100 pounds lighter, she could once again fit into the size-14 dress – this time with room to spare.

Now, her wardrobe contains only one larger-size garment, which she keeps around so she'll stay inspired to maintain her present weight of 10st 5lb. It's the size-26 white dress that she wore in that graduation photo.

WINNING ACTION ➤ ➤ ➤

Measure your progress with your wardrobe. Keep one article of clothing handy that will fit when you reach your ideal weight. Try it on from time to time to measure your progress. Use your try-on as motivation – and don't let yourself get depressed if it doesn't fit for weeks or months. Remember Dinah: the buttons on her black dress didn't close at first, but she persevered. Now, she has room to spare.

OLD PHOTO LED TO MOTHER AND DAUGHTER WEIGHT LOSS

They say that a picture is worth a thousand words. For Julia Ferraro and her mother, Adelaide, a photo is worth 90 pounds.

This particular photo, taken in June 1997, shows a father, mother, son and daughter, all smiling at their annual family picnic. It's a moment frozen in time, a vivid reminder of when Julia and Adelaide each weighed 14st 9lb. Both women are 5 foot 2 inches.

"Each of us got a copy of the picture for Christmas that year. My mum and I cried when we saw it. That was the fattest we had ever been," says Julia, 37. "You know you're getting bigger, but it doesn't really hit you until you look at a picture of yourself."

Instead of stashing the photo out of sight, Julia and Adelaide agreed to display it prominently in the front row of a table full of family photos. It gave them incentive to get serious about losing weight. Their first step was to join Weight Watchers the following February. Now, they attend classes every week.

Every day, Julia and Adelaide take a long look at that picnic photo. Since it was taken, the two women have lost a combined 90 pounds and five dress sizes. Julia, who's 50 pounds lighter, went from a size 20 to a 14. Her mother dropped 40 pounds, shrinking from a size 20 to a 16.

Both women want to lose more weight and they're pleased to report that they're well on their way. They've added a new photo to their tabletop gallery. This one shows a mother and daughter – slimmer and smiling.

WINNING ACTION ➤ ➤ ➤

Showcase your "before" photo. Find a photo of yourself and keep it where you can see it every day – on your bedside table or refrigerator, for example. As you lose weight, take new photos and display them with your old photo. They'll serve as visual reminders of where you started and where you're headed in terms of your weight-loss goals.

SHE GAVE 100 PER CENT AND LOST 115 POUNDS

As a personal trainer and motivational speaker, Barbara Press is devoting her life to helping others meet their health-and-fitness goals. To look at this dynamic young woman now, you'd never guess that she once weighed 17st 12lb.

"I turned my life around and I tell everyone who asks me that they can, too," she says. "But I also tell them that if they're not willing to give 100 per cent, they shouldn't even bother getting started."

It was her own willingness to give 100 per cent that transformed Barbara from an overweight, out-of-shape 20-year-old into the fit and trim 33-year-old that she is today. Her 115-pound weight loss was spurred by a man whom she barely knew.

"We were on our first – and last – date when, for reasons that

I still can't explain, he started telling me that I was too fat," she recalls. "At the time, I was hurt and angry. But his insults persuaded me to turn my life around. If I were to run into that guy today, I'd thank him from the bottom of my heart."

Once Barbara made up her mind to slim down, she went at it with gusto. "I worked harder at that than at anything that I ever had before," she says.

She read as much as she could on all aspects of weight loss, then began making changes in her diet. She concentrated on controlling her portion sizes and making healthy food choices. Within 1 year, she lost 60 pounds.

Inspired by her progress, Barbara added exercise to her weight-loss programme. She walked regularly, working her way up to 5 miles every day. "I got addicted to it," she says. "My day just wasn't complete without a good workout."

After taking off those first 60 pounds, Barbara set a more modest goal: to lose just 10 pounds a year. She consistently surpassed that goal and by 26, she had dropped to 9st 9lb.

One year later, after losing her job in the insurance industry, Barbara enlisted in the navy at her brother's urging. She served as a physical fitness coordinator for 6 years. "If I hadn't lost all of that weight, I never would have got into the military," she says. "Slimming down definitely changed my life."

During her stint in the navy, Barbara allowed her weight to bounce back to a more comfortable 11st 1lb, where she is still holding steady. These days, she's a full-time student, pursuing a bachelor's degree in health education. She works as a personal trainer at a local gym and has her own health-and-fitness business on the side. And she's often invited to speak about weight loss and health to various groups in her community.

When new clients visit Barbara for the first time, she asks them to spend a day or two thinking about whether they're ready to commit 100 per cent to a fitness programme. "I want them to understand that getting healthy isn't something that they can work at for a couple of days and then forget about for a while," she says. "Anybody can do a fitness programme and feel great. But you have to be ready to give what it takes."

> ## WINNING ACTION ➤➤➤
>
> **Contemplate your ability to commit.** Take Barbara's advice: spend a day or two carefully considering whether you're really ready to commit to eating better and exercising more. You may realise that now is not the time or that slimming down isn't a high priority for you or that you're doing it for the wrong reasons. As the first of the Ten Commandments of Weight Loss says, you have to believe in yourself and make yourself a top priority in order for weight loss to happen. When you're really ready, then nothing will stop you!

SHE SHED FAD DIETS AND 120 POUNDS

Laurie Slawta was the quintessential yo-yo dieter. She would lose weight – even as much as 40 pounds – only to have it come back again. But once she stopped dieting, she dropped 120 pounds. And they *haven't* come back.

"I tried every fad diet and diet pill known to woman," says Laurie, the 34-year-old wife of a dairy farmer. There was the grapefruit diet, the cabbage-soup diet, the high-protein, no-carbohydrate diet – you name it, she did it. But she lost more money than weight. She peaked at 20st 9lb.

Then, in August 1995, Laurie developed heel spurs. The pain was so overwhelming that she could barely walk. "I was told that an operation would take care of the spurs, but only temporarily," she says. "If I didn't lose weight, they'd come back."

Laurie knew that this meant permanent lifestyle changes.

The following month, she joined TOPS (Take Off Pounds Sensibly), where she learned how to make healthy, lower-calorie food choices. TOPS leaders also encouraged her to exercise. Her feet still throbbed from pain, so she purchased an inexpensive, non-impact exercise machine that simulates the movements of walking and stairclimbing.

Five months later, she was down 50 pounds and she switched to low-impact aerobics. By summer, she was down 5 stone and she started walking outside. By winter, the heel spurs were gone and so were 90 pounds. By March 1998, she achieved her goal weight of 12st 1lb.

Laurie has noticed other positive effects of slimming down. "I used to feel so exhausted that I'd fall asleep by 8 o'clock in the evening," she says. "Now, I have enough energy to carry me and my family through the day."

WINNING ACTION ➤ ➤ ➤

Don't fall for fad diets. As Laurie found out, there is no such thing as a miracle diet. Pills, potions and programmes that promise to take off a lot of weight in a little time sometimes work. The trouble is that the pounds almost always come back. For permanent weight loss, slow and steady wins the race.

SHE LOST 120 POUNDS ON HER OWN TERMS

After failing at a dozen different weight-loss plans, Lisa Douglass decided to create her own. "I just couldn't have someone telling me what I could or couldn't eat. I wanted to be responsible for my choices," she says. "I wanted absolute control."

Lisa, a computer analyst, bought a dozen exercise and nutrition videos. She studied books on food. She planned her workouts, meals and shopping trips. She kept a journal in which she noted how certain foods affected her weight and even her moods.

The plan she eventually created was healthy, sensible and geared to her eating habits and exercise interests. She decreased the amount of fat and sodium in her diet by preparing meals featuring lots of vegetables but very little red meat and by avoiding salty snacks and fast food. "Because I was choosing foods that were healthier and lower in calories, I didn't really have to limit my portion sizes," she notes. She also started working out on a treadmill, gradually working up to 1-hour runs, 5 or 6 days a week. Her plan worked. Over 2 years, Lisa dropped from 20 stone to 11st 6lb.

"I'm 5 foot 7 inches, so I carry my weight well. People tell me I look good," she says. "Still, I'd like to drop another 10 to 15 pounds."

Lisa, now 29, believes she needs a new plan to take off those last few stubborn pounds. She's experimenting with changes in her diet and exercise routines, but concedes that it has been a battle to stay focused. "Sometimes I make good choices, sometimes bad," she says. "But I like the fact that I'm the one making the choices."

WINNING ACTION ➤ ➤ ➤

Design the perfect plan for you. No one weight-loss plan fits all. The best is a hand-picked hotchpotch of personal secrets and strategies. To make your own, expose yourself to a variety of sources: books, classes, groups like Weight Watchers or TOPS (Take Off Pounds Sensibly), even nutritionists and personal trainers. Take the best from each and stick with what works for you.

SHE HAS A PLAN FOR STAYING SLIM

Sharon Duke leaves nothing to chance. She meticulously plans out every detail of every day – from when and what she eats to where and how she exercises, from trips to the shops to trips out of town.

That may seem like a lot of work. But Sharon, 51, doesn't want to leave anything to chance, especially in terms of maintaining a healthy weight.

What spurred this painstaking attention to detail? As her fiftieth birthday approached, Sharon noticed that her weight had crept up to 11st 7lb – too much for her 5-foot-3-inch frame. She had been gaining a couple of pounds every year since her mid-forties. Because she ate healthily and exercised regularly, she didn't think that her lifestyle was to blame for the 35 extra pounds. Instead, she suspected that the combination of advancing age and menopause were stalling her metabolism.

Sharon decided that she'd have to be even more vigilant about her healthy lifestyle if she wanted to bring back her slim and shapely figure. "At the time, my health club was offering a 6-week nutrition-awareness class, so I signed up," Sharon recalls. "I discovered that even though I was making good food choices, I was eating far too much. That's what got me started on planning ahead."

If she had a business lunch with colleagues, she found out in advance where they intended to eat and chose her meal beforehand. "I'd call the restaurant and ask if they offered a salad with grilled chicken or a fruit salad," she says. "If they didn't have what I wanted, I'd eat before we went out, then just order a side salad at the restaurant."

When her job required her to travel out of town, she called restaurants near where she was staying and enquired about their menus. "If I couldn't find one with suitable menu items, I'd go to a shop and pick up some food to take back to my room," she says.

Sharon applied her plan-ahead strategy to her exercise

programme, too. Before she travelled, she called the hotel to find out whether it had exercise equipment or if there was a gym nearby. If not, during her hotel stay she got up early to take a 2-mile walk or she climbed stairs at the hotel.

Once she started mapping out her daily routine, Sharon lost the extra 35 pounds within 6 months. She has maintained her weight at 9 stone since 1998.

WINNING ACTION ➤ ➤ ➤

Prepare a daily plan. If you find yourself struggling to stick with your weight-loss programme, Sharon's strategy may work for you, too. You may even want to keep a daily planner, which you can buy in any stationer's store. Then each night, spend 15 minutes or so mapping out the next day. Include as much detail as you can, especially in terms of mealtimes and workout time. Of course, you can't always anticipate what will happen every moment of every day. But a daily plan gives you a better chance of keeping your weight-loss efforts on track.

WITH A PASSPORT, SHE DISCOVERED A HEALTHIER LIFESTYLE

Barb Rand never thought much about her lifestyle until she spent a year in Kuala Lumpur, Malaysia. There, she discovered how a simpler life could help her slim down.

While a newspaper reporter in a big American city, Barb had grown fond of a typical Western diet – especially the huge cuts of beef served in steakhouses and the barbecued chicken and ribs. Because she was fairly active, playing tennis and jogging on occasion, her waistline didn't suffer as much as it could have. Still, she eventually carried 9st 4lb on her 5-foot-5-inch frame and she

was used to being a lot leaner. Then, cued by her social con-
science, Barb signed on as a volunteer abroad with a non-profit
organisation. Her assignment took her to Kuala Lumpur, where she
was to help local women start their own businesses.

Once she arrived, she couldn't help but notice the vast dif-
ferences between Malaysia and the United States, especially in
terms of diet and lifestyle.

In Malaysia, for example, beef isn't an everyday food. It's used
only sparingly in special-occasion dishes. Eggs and processed
foods are also rarities. Instead, Malaysians eat rice or noodles
topped with small helpings of stir-fry or curry. They also enjoy a
rich array of native fruits, including bananas, starfruit and bright
red, spiny rambutans.

Barb embraced the traditional Malaysian diet. She found that
she could eat as much as she wanted without widening her waistline. And she walked almost everywhere. By the time she came
home a year later, she discovered that she had dropped 20 pounds
without even trying.

"It was easy to lose weight in Malaysia because of the normal
lifestyle," Barb says. "It made me realise how excessive we are in the
West. We regularly eat huge portions of foods that are considered
luxuries in other parts of the world. And we drive everywhere. In
Malaysia, people walk a lot more."

Upon returning home in 1988, Barb resolved not to gain back
the weight that she had lost. So she incorporated much of what she
had learned in Malaysia into her lifestyle. To this day, she eats lots of
grains but very few meats, eggs or dairy products. She tries to buy fresh,
organically grown produce whenever possible and has cut down on
processed foods. She even planted a vegetable garden so she could
raise some of her food on her own. For exercise, she resumed jogging and she plays tennis and basketball with her 7-year-old son.

Since adopting a simpler, healthier lifestyle, Barb has had no trouble keeping off those 20 pounds. At 43, she maintains her weight at 7st 12lb. "I have a lot more energy, too," she says.

> ## WINNING ACTION ➤ ➤ ➤
>
> **Bring a global perspective to your weight-loss efforts.** It's ironic, isn't it? We are surrounded by so much prosperity that we spend a fortune on losing weight. Take a tip from other cultures and look for ways to simplify your life. Build your meals around foods that you could grow yourself – grains, vegetables and fruits. Reserve meats and dairy products for special occasions. (In fact, the Asian Food Pyramid limits meats to just one serving per month!) And whenever possible, leave your car in the garage and walk or cycle to your destination. You'll get thinner and you'll probably live longer, too.

THE SECRET IS OUT:
SHE'S 5 STONE SLIMMER

Irma Toce travelled to America from Holland in 1987 – healthy, fit, trim and looking for adventure. Her goal was to work for 3 months, travel around the country and go back home. The reality was that she fell in love, got married and stayed in the United States.

And somewhere along the line, she gained 80 pounds.

While most of these dramatic life changes were a bit a of surprise, her weight gain was not. "I married into an Italian family that loves to eat," Irma says. "And I stopped walking as much as I used to in Holland."

By 1997, her weight had peaked at 17st 2lb. She was depressed, had no energy and hated what she saw in the mirror. It was a sharp contrast from who she was the decade before. "I couldn't believe what had happened to me," she says. "I knew that I had to do something and make a change. A big change."

With Dutch determination, she set her goal for 11st 6lb, her wedding-day weight. But she kept her plan a secret. "I stopped eating biscuits and started walking 5 days a week," she says. "I didn't tell anyone – not even my family."

Within 2 months, she lost 10 pounds. People noticed. Unable to hide her efforts, she confirmed "diet" speculations. "The support that I got was unbelievable," she says.

Clients and colleagues told Irma how wonderful she looked. And she finally started eating three meals a day. "Before, I would skip breakfast, then snack my way through the morning and afternoon, stopping only for lunch and dinner," she explains.

On sunny days when Irma didn't feel like exercising, her eldest stepdaughter would encourage her to take a walk. When chilly autumn weather provided another convenient excuse to skip her stroll, her husband bought her a treadmill.

Irma started to feel better about herself. Suddenly, everything changed for the better. "I even started to laugh at jokes again," she says.

Three years later, Irma was down to 12st 2lb. She's still 10 pounds shy of her goal, but she's confident that she'll hit her wedding-day weight soon. Her advice to others who want to slim down is, "Stay positive and don't talk yourself down. If you blow it once in a while, get right back on track. Just take it one day at a time and don't be too hard on yourself. After all, you're worth it!"

WINNING ACTION ➤ ➤ ➤

Spread the word that you're trying to lose. According to a University of Pittsburgh study, those supported by friends and family have a 95 per cent chance of slimming down successfully. What's more, they are twice as likely to keep the extra pounds and inches off.

COUPLE DANCED AWAY 115 POUNDS

For better or worse, newlyweds Charlene and Eric Sutherland vowed to lose weight together. They just didn't anticipate how much fun it would be.

At a total of 34st 4lb – 14st 4lb for her, 20 stone for him – Charlene and Eric had resigned themselves to being hefty. "We'd been heavy all of our lives and diets never worked, so we stopped taking our weight problem seriously," Charlene recalls.

Still, as Christmas 1997 rolled around, the 24-year-old couple dreaded their families' weight-directed comments that were sure to come. So they bought a set of scales. Shocked by what they said, the couple felt that they *needed* to lose weight. This time, they would try exercise.

But a dilemma surfaced instantly. "We really wanted to do this together. We just didn't see eye-to-eye on how – not at first, anyway," Charlene says. "I like aerobics and lifting weights, but I hate gyms. I wanted to work out in front of the TV. But Eric gets bored. He's more of a sports guy."

Fortunately, the newlyweds found a creative compromise: dancing. In reminiscing about his dancing days with friends, Eric remembered that it had helped him to cut back his weight during his university days.

But neither Charlene nor Eric wanted to return to the smoky club scene, so they transformed their living room into a dance hall. Pushing aside the coffee table, the duo jammed to the fast-paced tunes of their favourite 1980s and 1990s bands for an hour every night.

"Dancing satisfied Eric's need to do something interesting and my need to avoid health clubs," Charlene explains. Their team approach worked so well that they decided to apply it to their eating habits. Together, they gave up junk food and fizzy drinks and they trimmed the fat content of their meals.

A year later and a collective 115 pounds lighter, this couple is ready to resize their wedding rings.

WINNING ACTION ➤ ➤ ➤

Drop pounds as a pair. If your spouse needs to slim down, too, why not do it together? It will be more fun and it may bring you even closer together. Dancing is an ideal activity for couples, but if it doesn't appeal to you or your spouse, find something that you both like. Compare lists of your favourite activities or browse class offerings at your local leisure centre or health club to see if something piques your and your spouse's interest.

FAMILY OF THREE LOST 150 POUNDS

Jane Brennan's family lost an entire person.

Not literally, of course. But between the three of them – 56-year-old Jane, her 57-year-old husband, Bob and their 29-year-old daughter, Jennifer – they've taken off more than 150 pounds. They've done it by turning weight loss into a family affair, according to Jane.

It all started when Jane finally gave in to her daughter's constant nagging to do something, anything, to slim down. Jane had put on about 60 pounds over the course of 17 years, going from a size 12 to an 18. And Jennifer seemed to be following in her mother's footsteps, going from a size 10 to a size 18.

Together, mother and daughter went to Weight Watchers. As they started losing weight, Jane's husband decided to get in on the act. Over the years, Bob's own waistline had expanded from 38 inches to 42.

The threesome were determined to take off and keep off the extra pounds. Every day, they compared notes about what they had eaten and how much. They exchanged ideas for keeping their eating habits on track – for example, munching on carrot sticks to fill up. As often as possible, they ate meals together. "No one was moaning and groaning, especially about what we had for dinner," Jane says. "All of us had the same goal. We talked the same language."

For Jane, who had tried to lose weight in the past, having the support of her family made all the difference. "I think there's a definite advantage to losing weight with other people, especially those who share your eating times and rituals," she says. "That way, you can encourage each other. You might have a bit of friendly competition, too."

> ### WINNING ACTION ➤➤➤
>
> **Get your family involved.** Ask everyone in your household to join you in your weight-loss efforts. When the entire family participates, meal planning becomes much easier. Plus, family members can support, encourage and inspire one another.

HER CALENDAR KEEPS HER TRUE TO HER DIET

To keep your weight-loss programme on the right track, dangling motivational carrots in front of your nose can help. Just ask Bevan Brooks, a legislative aide and a successful weight-loss champion.

Right out of college, at 22, Bevan found herself heavier than she'd ever been. Not one to let such problems go unattended, she decided to make some lifestyle changes to help herself slim down and stay healthy. "I knew that it would be easier to do while I was still in my early twenties than when I got older," she says.

Without forcing herself into a rigid diet or exercise plan, she began eating better and working out regularly. She took up jogging and cut out addictive pepperoni pizzas. Over the course of a year, Bevan lost 20 pounds without counting fat grams, calories or even stepping on the scales very often. How, then, did she keep motivated?

"I would remind myself of activities and special events that were on my calendar in the weeks or months ahead," Bevan says. She liked the idea of looking her best and being in good enough shape for whatever was coming her way. Parties, trips, sporting events, visitors from out of town and other occasions in the not-too-distant future were fuel for her commitment.

She knew that she wanted to look good for her best friend's beach wedding, for example. Every time she thought about missing a workout or eating too much pepperoni pizza, Bevan would remind herself about the wedding. She rarely strayed. "How I looked meant more to me than a pepperoni pizza," she says.

Today, if her schedule looks jam-packed one week, Bevan makes sure that she doesn't miss any workouts or healthy meals the week before. That way, during her busy week she can skip a run or eat something a bit richer than normal during a stressful day without beating herself up about it.

"Knowing what's on my calendar also helps me get up to work out in the morning, especially if I know that I might go out with friends after work," she adds.

WINNING ACTION ➤➤➤

Check your calendar for weight-loss "carrots". Instead of just focusing on reaching a certain size or shape, keep your motivational focus fresh. Use an upcoming occasion as incentive to work out and eat right. Then, once it has passed, check your diary for the next big event.

SHE LOST THE WEIGHT
AND GOT HER DREAM JOB

Phyllis Schmoyer wanted to be a telephone operator, just like her big sister. So shortly after leaving school in 1944, she applied for a job at the same company where her sister worked.

"At first, I was told that I couldn't be hired because it was against company policy to employ more than one person from the same family," recalls the 73 year old. "But when I pressed the issue, I was told that I was too heavy." At the time, she carried 12 stone on her 5-foot-5-inch frame.

"Back then, telephone operators sat very close to one another," she explains. "Because I was overweight, I would have taken up more than my share of space."

Phyllis, who had never been too concerned about her weight, suddenly had a very compelling reason to slim down. "I really wanted that job, so I began doing things that I thought would help me get rid of the extra pounds," she recalls. "I stopped sitting around like I had done all during school and I started walking everywhere." She also tried to eat better, cutting back on both the sweets that she loved and the rich food that was served in her home. "I was accustomed to heavy meals with lots of fried foods," she says.

Sure enough, the pounds came off – 40 of them in all. Triumphant, Phyllis returned to the phone company to reapply for an operator position. This time, she got the job.

Though more than 50 years have passed, Phyllis has maintained her trim figure. "I stay active and I watch what I eat," she says. "I think that my weight got to where it was supposed to be in the first place and it has pretty much stayed there."

Looking back, Phyllis is convinced that taking off those 40 pounds made a world of difference for her. "If I hadn't lost the weight, I probably wouldn't be alive today," she says. "Heart disease runs in my family and as heavy as I was, I might have got it, too. I truly believe that slimming down saved my life."

WINNING ACTION ➤ ➤ ➤

Make slimming down high stakes. If you have trouble sticking with your weight-loss programme, maybe you need to up the ante a bit. Maybe you've been toying with the idea of changing jobs or going back to school or signing up for an African safari. Make that your incentive to slim down.

NEVER TOO OLD TO LOSE

Connie Bissonnette had all but given up on slimming down. Aged 50 and 12st 4lb, the full-time university lecturer believed that weight gain was a normal part of the ageing process.

Luckily for her, her son Jeff knew better. And as a result of his persistence, Connie is 41 pounds thinner.

In 1992, Jeff was at university, studying human performance. When he came home for Christmas break that year, he had a mission: to persuade his mum to start exercising. "I was his first project," Connie jokes.

She responded with her usual litany of excuses – she didn't have time, she didn't have the energy, her knees bothered her. But Jeff persisted. "He said, 'Just give me 10 minutes, three times a week,'" Connie recalls. "He devised a workout that I could do at home, with what I had on hand. I started out by sitting in a chair and doing leg lifts. Then I added other exercises, like doing pushups against the wall."

Despite her initial protests, Connie found herself enjoying her workout. Within a few months, she noticed that her knees felt better. So she asked Jeff to add some more exercises to her routine. Her 10-minute exercise sessions stretched to as long as 30 minutes.

Plus, she started walking for 30 minutes, 2 or 3 days a week. One year later, she was 20 pounds lighter.

But Jeff wasn't done. His next challenge was to transform his mother's longtime meat-and-potatoes diet. Again, he advised Connie to start small. She substituted jam for butter on her morning toast, fresh fruit for her snack time crisps and sweets. Eventually, she traded frying for baking as her cooking method of choice.

It took some time, but all those little changes added up. Four years after she began exercising, Connie had lost a total of 41 pounds. Now, at 58, she has maintained her weight at about 9st 5lb since 1996.

Connie was so grateful to her son for helping her slim down that she decided to return the favour. In May 1997, she became a certified personal trainer. Now, she works in her son's gym. "It's great to be able to encourage the clients I train by telling them about my own weight-loss experience," she reports. "I don't let anyone say, 'I can't.'"

WINNING ACTION ➤ ➤ ➤

Stop believing the myth of middle-age spread. Yes, most of us do gain weight as the birthdays roll by. But this accumulation of extra pounds isn't written in our genes, our hormones or the laws of nature. We gain weight, quite simply, because we become less active. According to experts, about 80 per cent of weight gain is caused by a sedentary lifestyle. So keep moving, no matter what your age. You'll look slimmer and you'll feel younger.

SHE JUMPED OUT OF THE GENE POOL

For Cindy Engle, a family reunion ended a 14-year pattern of losing and regaining weight – and helped her permanently part with 20 pounds.

Like both of her parents, Cindy had struggled with her weight for most of her life. From the time she was in her late twenties, she tried just about everything to slim down. "I followed far too many diet plans. I took diet pills. I even ran half-marathons," says the 42-year-old mother of two. "Sure, I'd lose weight. But the pounds would always come back."

In the summer of 1998, Cindy attended the fateful family gathering. "When I looked around, I noticed that everyone had gained 5 to 10 pounds – maybe more – since the year before," she says. "That day, I made a serious commitment to losing weight."

Cindy wasn't about to accept what seemed like her genetic destiny. Because she already led a fairly active lifestyle, she decided to focus on revamping her eating habits. After reading up on nutrition, she began building her meals around fresh, nutritious foods: fruit for breakfast, salads and lean proteins for lunch and lean meats for dinner. She also began drinking lots of water – at least eight full glasses a day.

Within 4 months of making these simple dietary changes, Cindy had taken off 20 pounds. She has maintained her weight at a healthy 8st 5lb ever since, thanks to her dietary vigilance and her commitment to jogging 40 to 60 minutes, three or four times a week.

WINNING ACTION ➤ ➤ ➤

Reject the family fat gene. Do your relatives – especially parents, grandparents, aunts and uncles – struggle with their weight? If so, you may have a genetic predisposition towards being overweight. That doesn't mean you should accept it. Studies show that your lifestyle choices – what you eat and how much you exercise – are far more important than your genes in determining your weight.

THE SCALES STOOD
BETWEEN HER AND SUCCESS

Kym Hubert lost 85 pounds, but not until she finally threw out the scales that had become her obsession.

Kym had struggled with her weight for 20 years – a consequence of her preference for fatty foods (chocolate milkshakes were her favourite). In 1991, she joined a weight-loss programme that required daily weigh-ins. After 4 months, she dropped out, discouraged. But she didn't get rid of the scales.

Soon, Kym was weighing herself three times a day: in the morning after she got out of the shower (to see if she had lost weight overnight), before dinner (to see if she had lost weight during the day) and before bed (to see if she had gained weight during dinner). Unfortunately, her scales seldom showed good news. By June 1997, she weighed 17st 7lb.

Desperate to help Kym overcome her obsession with her weight, her husband smashed her scales. At first, she felt exasperated and frustrated. "It was sort of like having your addiction taken away from you," she says. "I became very depressed about my weight." But eventually, she was able to refocus her energy on a new interest: walking.

"My husband, who's a runner, belongs to a group that includes runners and walkers. He kept asking me to join the walkers in the group," she recalls. "I finally decided that I could either sit around and stay depressed or try something that might bring my husband and me closer together."

On her first outing with the walkers, Kym trekked 1½ miles. She hurt afterwards, but she agreed to meet the group the following Saturday. Pretty soon, she was also walking 3 nights a week, either with her husband or a girlfriend.

By April 1998, Kym felt fit enough to add running to her fitness programme. In October of that year, she joined a gym and weighed herself for the first time in months. She had lost 80 pounds, thanks largely to walking and running. And, as a bonus, she says, "My relationship with my husband has improved 1,000 per cent. We're spending more time together and I'm not feeling depressed anymore."

Today, at 41, Kym is more concerned about how she looks and feels than how much she weighs. She'll never again use scales to measure her success.

WINNING ACTION ➤ ➤ ➤

Stay off your scales. When you're trying to slim down, don't rely on your scales to measure your success. Because muscle is heavier than fat, your weight may not change much as you become more fit. Instead, some experts recommend using your clothes as a guide. Do your shirts and trousers feel looser? Do you have more room in the waist? If so, celebrate. That's the sign that you're making progress.

SHE MEASURES HER SUCCESS IN INCHES, NOT POUNDS

Rita Wolberg traded in her scales for a tape measure. It helped her slim down not once, but twice.

When she was 31, Rita, a computer program analyst, decided to join Weight Watchers to unload some extra pounds that had accumulated over the years. "I just overate and I didn't know what I should eat to be slim," she explains. She followed the programme to the letter, taking off 22 pounds in 12 weeks.

After the birth of her son some 5 years later, Rita developed chronic sinus infections. Four sinus surgeries later, she found that she had gained 30 pounds. "I had put on so much weight that I moved up 3 clothing sizes," she says. She went back to Weight Watchers and this time, she took off 30 pounds in 18 months. "I wasn't quite as vigilant about sticking with the programme," she admits. "I knew it would work. I just had to be patient."

On both occasions, Rita used a tape measure – not scales – to monitor her weight-loss progress. She found that by checking the circumference of her bust, waist, hips and thighs once a week, she had a more accurate record of her changing body shape. "Even the second time, when the pounds came off slowly, I could count on my tape measure to show that I was improving," she says. "Some part of my body was getting smaller, even if the scales didn't show it."

Rita, 45, now serves as a programme leader for Weight Watchers. "I started there as a receptionist in 1988 and they let me stay even when I regained weight," she says. "That really inspired me to want to spread their message." And she never misses an opportunity to tell others how valuable a tape measure can be as a weight-loss motivator.

WINNING ACTION ➤ ➤ ➤

Trade your scales for a tape measure. Scales won't tell you how your body composition has changed, but a tape measure can. As you lose fat and gain muscle, certain body parts get smaller. To check the size of your waist, wrap the tape around the narrowest part of your waist, roughly halfway between your bottom ribs and your hipbones. For your hips, wrap the tape around your hips and bottom at their widest points, usually slightly below the actual hipbones. Write down your measurements, then track them from week to week.

SHE LOST 125 POUNDS, 5 POUNDS AT A TIME

Susan DeFusco knows how to lose 100 pounds. She's done it twice. Only now she knows she has the formula right.

The first time she topped 14st 4lb was at school. "At the time, I had a jealous boyfriend," Susan says. "We didn't socialise much. In fact, about all we did was eat out. I think my overeating was a means of compensating for a lack of interaction with other people."

When she was 19 years old, she stopped getting her periods. Her doctor told her that it was because she was so overweight. This was the wake-up call that Susan needed. Once she made up her mind to slim down, she cut her weight by almost half in 1 year. "I did it mostly by changing my eating habits and giving up certain fattening foods," she says. "The trouble was, I never changed my *attitude* towards food. So once the weight was gone, my old eating habits returned."

A decade later, with two kids and bills to pay, Susan went over 200 pounds again. "I wasn't making the right choices food-wise and I wasn't exercising like I should have been," she says. "I can put on weight very quickly and it came back fast."

By 1994, Susan weighed 18st 8lb. Her back hurt so badly that she had trouble walking, let alone playing with her kids out in the garden. It was time to lose weight again.

While her overall goal was to shed 100 pounds, from day to day she focused only on losing the next 5. Each time she met one of her mini-goals, she rewarded herself with a small treat, like a bubble bath or an exercise tape.

"To wait until you get to your goal to say 'I'm going to treat myself' is too long a time," she says. "You need to look at each 5 pounds as something worth celebrating because it's closer and closer to where you want to be."

After a year and a few months of sensible eating, exercising and participating in the support group TOPS (Take Off Pounds Sensibly), Susan had met all of her little goals. They added up to 100 pounds – gone for good.

Inspired by her weight loss and religious about her exercise, Susan became a fitness instructor. And she lost another 25 pounds.

Now in her late thirties, Susan passes along her success story to her support group and at the fitness centre where she works. "It gives people hope," she says. "They realise that if I did it, they can do it."

WINNING ACTION ➤➤➤

Take small steps towards your big goals. Break down your weight-loss goal into 5-pound targets. Every time you hit one of those targets, celebrate. Write down a list of non-food treats – a pedicure, a massage, a new CD – and reward yourself every mini-step of the way.

A BAG OF SUGAR IS HER MEASURE OF SUCCESS

Whenever Pat Beyer gets the urge to splurge, she picks up a 5-pound bag of sugar.

"Five pounds of sugar is heavy," says Pat, 41. "When I think that I lost the equivalent of five of those bags, it's easy for me to resist temptation."

Pat found the extra 25 pounds after giving birth to twins in 1992. Three months later, she found the motivation to get rid of them when she saw a family photo. "I stood out in the photo, but not because of my outfit," she recalls.

A size 16 and only 5 foot 4 inches, Pat knew that she had to make a change. She joined Weight Watchers in October and was down to a size 10 at her twins' christening the following February.

Pat has successfully kept off her weight, but not without temptation. She has that bag of sugar as a reminder of what she used to weigh. "I remember coming back from the shops one day and lifting that 5-pound bag of sugar to put it in the cupboard," she says. "I thought, 'I lost five times that much!'"

That realisation has rescued Pat from many a sticky dietary situation over the years. She recalls one incident in 1998, when she was feeling particularly frazzled. "The kids hadn't eaten and they had to be at tennis and football practice on the opposite sides of town," she says. "I figured that the easiest thing was just to stop at McDonald's on the way." As she reached for her keys, she remembered the sugar. "I'd taken off five bags of sugar and I didn't want to add one back on," Pat says. She put down the keys and went to the kitchen to prepare a quick meal of chicken and vegetables.

WINNING ACTION ➤ ➤ ➤

Pick up a bag of sugar. Find a symbol of your weight loss – a 5-pound bag of sugar, a can of drink or a slab of bacon. When somebody suggests fast food, think about your symbol. Pick it up to remind yourself of how far you've come and how much additional weight you'd have to carry around if you gained it back.

HIS WAISTLINE SHRANK BY HALF

Ask John Therkelsen how he feels since he lost 189 pounds and he'll tell you that he is healthier, has more energy and has a brighter outlook on life. It's these sorts of positive changes – not just the decreasing number on the scales – that kept him on track for weight-loss success.

"Had I focused only on how many pounds I was taking off, I don't think I would have remained as strong and determined as I did," says 53-year-old John. "What kept me going was how good I felt and how much more I could do."

John had been heavy for most of his life. But his love of sports kept him active – until he developed plantar fasciitis, a painful foot condition, in 1996. Suddenly, he found himself sidelined, unable to golf, bowl, play tennis or engage in other activities that he had always enjoyed. In the 2 years that it took his foot to heal, his weight climbed to 26 stone. By that time, he was so out of shape that he couldn't resume his active lifestyle.

Realising that he was dangerously obese and that he needed help to slim down, John researched several weight-loss facilities before settling on one. "A colleague had recommended it to me and several health-care providers whom I know personally gave it their thumbs-up," he says. He signed up for an 8-week residential programme, during which he learned about the three major components of weight loss: nutrition, exercise and the psychological aspects of food and eating.

The education and support that he received enabled John to lose 4 stone during the 8-week programme. Once he returned home, he continued to follow the eating plan and to track his calorie intake. He made visits to a local gym and looked for ways to increase the amount of activity in his daily routine, like walking to work or to the grocery store. He also eased back into the sports he loved – tennis, golf and skiing.

As determined as he was to slim down, John understood that he had a long way to go before he reached a healthy weight. To keep himself motivated, he looked for other markers of his progress. And he found plenty: his increasing strength and stamina from regular exercise, his lower blood pressure and cholesterol readings, his more positive attitude. "Watching all of these things improve provided tremendous motivation for me," he says. "It really kept me encouraged."

By spring 1999, a little more than a year after starting his weight-loss programme, John stabilized at 12st 7lb. His waist measurement shrank from 60 inches to 34, reducing his clothing size from a XXL to a medium. Needless to say, he's fitter, healthier and feeling better than ever.

John will be the first to tell you that slimming down takes time and commitment. "But so many positive changes occur along the way," he says. "Look at these other accomplishments as part of your success, even if weight loss is your ultimate goal."

WINNING ACTION ➤ ➤ ➤

Find inspiration along the way. Lasting weight loss is a slow and steady process. Instead of focusing on how many pounds you've lost, look for other changes in your health, appearance and attitude. Has your blood pressure gone down? Do your clothes fit better? Do you feel more energetic and alive? Acknowledge and enjoy these accomplishments. They prove that you're doing all the right things to achieve weight-loss success.

---

400 POUNDS
GONE – AND COUNTING

Since 1992, Linda Matulin has lost 400 pounds, a full two-thirds of her body weight. The 44 year old attributes her success to discipline, determination and one well-timed television show.

At her heaviest, Linda carried more than 42st 12lb on her 5-foot-6-inch frame. "I don't remember a time in my life when I wasn't overweight," she says. "But I really started to gain when I got a job working a night shift. I don't know why, but I ate all the time."

Linda went on and off diets, never making much progress in her battle of the bulge. "Maybe that's because I never tried really hard," she says. "It may be difficult to believe, but I never saw myself as fat, even at 600 pounds. I lived a full life, doing everything I wanted – socialising with friends, going to concerts, travelling."

Her mindset abruptly changed on the day that she happened to catch a television interview with country singer Lorrie Morgan. "The interview had nothing to do with weight loss or fitness. Lorrie was talking about herself and her life – how she took control and made changes," Linda recalls. "For me, something clicked. I became absolutely convinced that this time, I could really lose the weight."

Despite her excitement, Linda said nothing to her family. "I knew that they meant well, but I didn't want their advice," she says. "The people closest to you tend to put a lot of pressure on you when you're dieting." She'd been through all that many times before, when she had tried different diets – and failed.

On her own, Linda began making dramatic lifestyle changes that supported her weight-loss goals. Most important, she stopped eating on autopilot, instead letting her body tell her when it needed food and how much. "It had always been telling me these things," she says. "I just never took the time to listen."

Having grown accustomed to eating as much as she wanted, whenever she wanted, Linda found the going to be tough at first. She had days when she devoured almost anything in sight. "But the more I focused on my body's hunger signals, the less food – especially fatty food – appealed to me," she says. And that's when she started to lose weight.

Linda also looked for ways to be more active during the day. She started with some gentle movements in her swimming pool. After she dropped some pounds, she graduated to working out on a treadmill. "I'd do what I felt like doing on a particular day," she says. "I didn't have a set exercise plan, but I tried to move around a lot."

Even as she lost weight, Linda continued to conceal her trimmer physique under her newly baggy clothes. "I remained reluctant to tell my family what I was up to because I didn't want them offering me advice," she explains. When she finally broke down and bought some smaller-size clothing, she wowed even those closest to her. "They were surprised, to say the least," she says. "But they were really happy for me, too."

Today, Linda is literally a shadow of her former self. In the years since she first began her weight-loss programme, she has dropped 400 pounds to 14st 4lb. She hopes to get down to 12st 7lb, a goal that is certainly within her reach.

"Sometimes, I get a little frustrated because I'm not there yet," she says. "But then I remind myself that I didn't lose 400 pounds overnight. I'll achieve my goal in good time."

WINNING ACTION ➤ ➤ ➤

Remember that you can do it. Linda's story is an important inspiration for all of us. No matter how much weight you want to lose, even if it's 400 pounds, you can succeed. It may take some time – but remember, if Linda could do it, so can you.